ENGLISH EXPRESSIONS IN CONTEXT

Medical edition

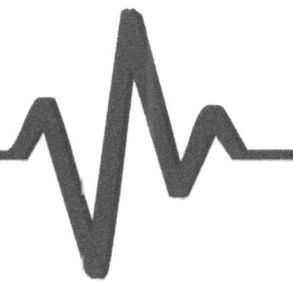

Natacha Lazareff
and Ken Takahashi

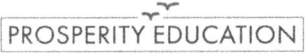

Registered offices: Sherlock Close, Cambridge
CB3 0HP, United Kingdom

First published 2025

ISBN: 978-1-915654-36-6

© Prosperity Education Ltd. 2025

This publication is in copyright. Subject to statutory exception and to the provisions of relevant collective licensing agreements, no reproduction of any part may take place without the written permission of Prosperity Education.

The moral rights of the authors have been asserted.

Designed by ORP Cambridge

For further information and resources, visit:
www.prosperityeducation.net

To infinity and beyond.

Contents

Introduction   *4*

accommodate (vt)	8	deficient (adj)	42	infer (vt)	76
acquiesce (vi)	9	defy (vt)	43	inherent (adj)	77
advocate (vt, vi, n)	10	deplete (vt)	44	integral (adj)	78
affect (vt)	11	deviate (vi)	45	interrogate (vt)	79
aggravate (vt)	12	diminish (vi, vt)	46	intriguing (adj)	80
aggregate (vt, adj)	13	discern (vt)	47	intrinsic (adj)	81
anecdotal (adj)	14	disparity (n)	48	invoke (vt)	82
anomaly (n)	15	disrupt (vt)	49	manifest (vt, vi, adj)	83
appraise (vt)	16	distort (vt)	50	mitigate (vt)	84
attenuate (vt)	17	diverge (vi)	51	mundane (adj)	85
battered (adj)	18	efficacy (n)	52	myriad (n, adj)	86
benevolent (adj)	19	efficient (adj)	53	perceive (vt)	87
bolster (vt)	20	elicit (vt)	54	postulate (vi, vt)	88
circumvent (vi)	21	eliminate (vt)	55	potent (adj)	89
cognitive (adj)	22	empirical (adj)	56	premise (n, vt)	90
compensate (vi)	23	endure (vt, vi)	57	proliferate (vi)	91
compound (vt)	24	enhance (vt)	58	prove (vt)	92
concede (vt, vi)	25	ensue (vi)	59	provoke (vt)	93
concurrent (adj)	26	equitable (adj)	60	ramp up (phrV)	94
conducive (adj)	27	eradicate (vt)	61	regimen (n)	95
confer (vt, vi)	28	erroneous (adj)	62	remit (vi, vt)	96
congruent (adj)	29	exacerbate (vt)	63	resolve (vt, vi)	97
conjure (vi, vt)	30	extract (vt, n)	64	robust (adj)	98
consistent (adj)	31	explicit (adj)	65	sentient (adj)	99
consolidate (vt, vi)	32	extrapolate (vi, vt)	66	speculate (vi, vt)	100
contradict (vt, vi)	33	feasible (adj)	67	stagnate (vi)	101
contravene (vt)	34	firsthand (adj, adv)	68	strenuous (adj)	102
corroborate (vt)	35	heterogeneous (adj)	69	succumb (vi)	103
credible (adj)	36	homogeneous (adj)	70	sustain (vt)	104
culminate (vi)	37	impair (vt)	71	underscore (vt)	105
cumulative (adj)	38	imperative (adj)	72	understate (vt)	106
debilitate (vt)	39	implicit (adj)	73	uphold (vt)	107
deduce (vt)	40	incremental (adj)	74	visceral (adj)	108
deem (vt)	41	induce (vt)	75		

Endmatter   *110*

Introduction

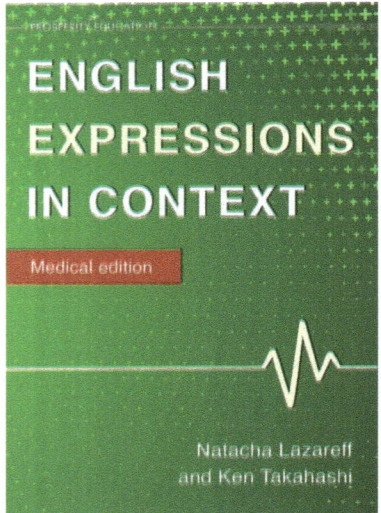

This book is not merely a compilation of vocabulary or a review of grammar. Rather, it presents **101 carefully selected lexical items** chosen for their frequency and relevance in professional medical contexts. Lexical knowledge alone does not guarantee effective communication, so to achieve a high level of proficiency it is essential to understand how words combine naturally — through *collocations* — and to use them appropriately within context to convey meaning with precision and nuance.

This principle lies at the heart of *English Expressions in Context: Medical Edition*. The resource is designed to equip intermediate-to-advanced users of English with the linguistic tools required to communicate clearly, accurately and confidently in clinical, academic and professional medical settings.

A practical guide to mastering medical English

Unlike general English resources, this book features authentic, domain-specific dialogues and textual excerpts that reflect genuine communicative situations encountered in medical practice — ranging from patient consultations and interdisciplinary meetings to conference presentations and formal documentation. This context-driven approach recognises that healthcare professionals must master a register of English that extends well beyond every-day conversation, encompassing specialised terminology, complex collocational patterns and the discourse conventions characteristic of professional and scientific communication.

Intended audience

This resource is designed for healthcare practitioners including physicians, nurses, allied health professionals and researchers working in medicine, public health and related disciplines. It is particularly valuable for candidates preparing for **the Occupational English Test (OET)**. The interactive dialogues closely parallel OET speaking scenarios, the clinical documentation models (such as referral letters, discharge summaries and transfer notes) align with OET writing tasks, and the inclusion of academic extracts enhances the advanced reading skills essential for examination success.

About the authors

This publication represents a long-standing collaboration between **Dr Ken Takahashi** (MD, MPH, PhD), an internationally recognised authority in occupational health, and **Natacha Lazareff** (MA, MSc, SEPiT, TEFL) a linguistic coach specialising in professional language development. Their partnership brings together extensive medical expertise and deep linguistic insight. Dr Takahashi's own experience — navigating English as a non-native professional under Ms Lazareff's guidance — provides an authentic foundation for this work. Together, they have produced a pedagogical resource grounded in both theory and lived experience, addressing the real communicative demands of healthcare professionals operating in English-speaking environments.

How to use this book

Each expression entry is carefully structured to support efficient and practical learning:

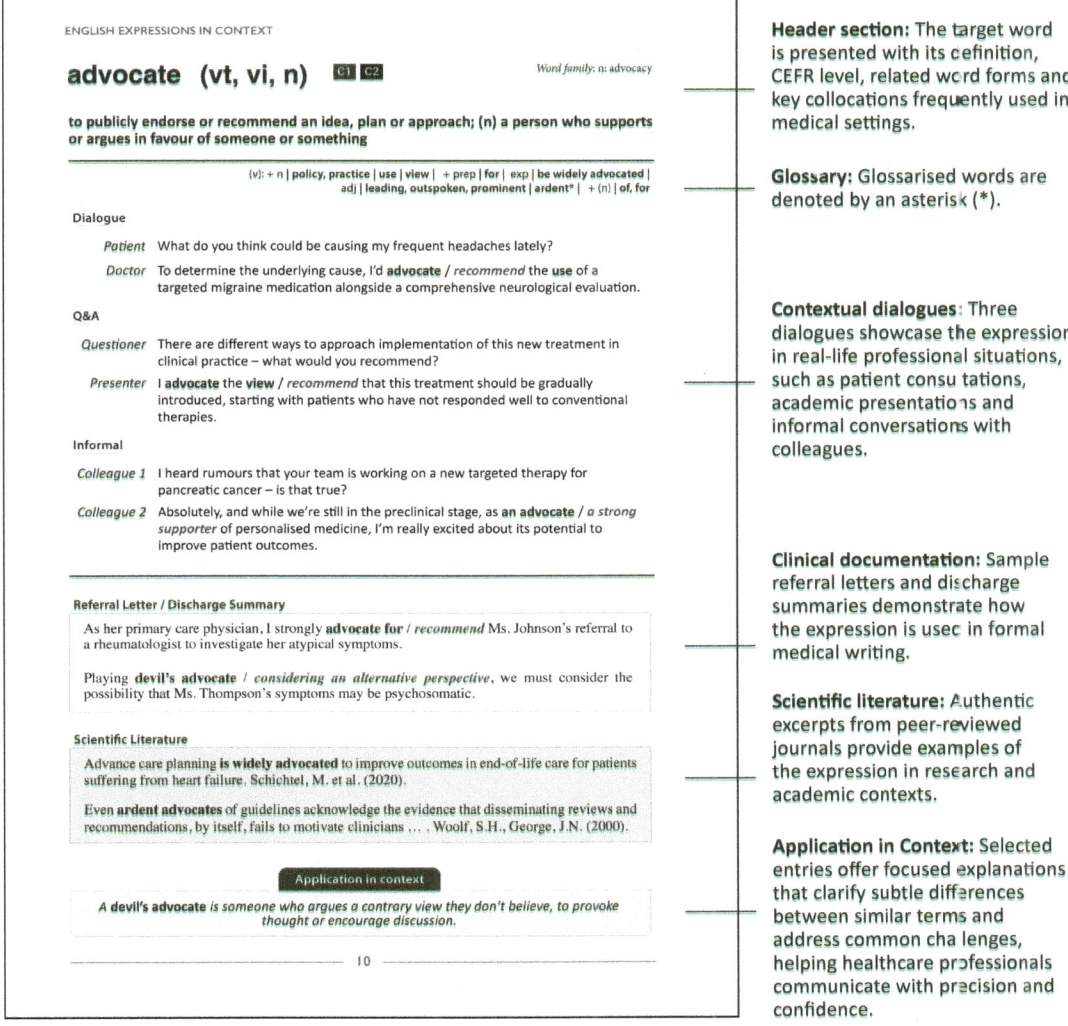

Header section: The target word is presented with its definition, CEFR level, related word forms and key collocations frequently used in medical settings.

Glossary: Glossarised words are denoted by an asterisk (*).

Contextual dialogues: Three dialogues showcase the expression in real-life professional situations, such as patient consultations, academic presentations and informal conversations with colleagues.

Clinical documentation: Sample referral letters and discharge summaries demonstrate how the expression is used in formal medical writing.

Scientific literature: Authentic excerpts from peer-reviewed journals provide examples of the expression in research and academic contexts.

Application in Context: Selected entries offer focused explanations that clarify subtle differences between similar terms and address common challenges, helping healthcare professionals communicate with precision and confidence.

At the end of the book (pages 110—120), you'll find valuable supplementary materials designed to deepen your understanding and support your ongoing learning journey.

- **Expanded Application in Context:** Several entries from the Application in Context sections are explored in greater detail here. This includes helpful comparison tables that clarify subtle differences between similar terms and address common-usage challenges faced by healthcare professionals.

- **Glossary of Terms:** A comprehensive glossary provides clear definitions of specialised medical terminology used throughout the book, making it easy to review and reinforce key concepts. Glossarised words are denoted by an asterisk (*).

- **Bibliography:** Full citations for all scientific literature excerpts featured in the text are listed here, allowing you to explore original research sources.

Expressions

The following abbreviations are used throughout this resource:
- adj: adjective
- adv: adverb
- ant: antonym
- coll: collocation
- exp: expression
- n: noun
- phrV: phrasal verb
- prep: preposition
- sub conj: subordinating conjunction
- syn: synonym
- vt: transitive verb
- vi: intransitive verb

accommodate (vt)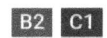

Word family: adj: accommodating, accommodative; n: accommodation

to consider opinions or facts when making decisions; to assist someone by fulfilling their request; to adjust behavior to adapt to a new situation

+ n as object | change | demand, request | needs

Dialogue

Patient   I'm worried about how my new work schedule might interfere with my treatment plan.

Doctor   Don't worry, we can adjust your appointment times to **accommodate** / *fit* your changing **needs**.

Q&A

Questioner   How do you plan to scale up your research to **accommodate** / *meet* the increasing **demand** for this new drug?

Presenter   We are exploring partnerships with larger research institutions to expand our capacity and resources.

Informal

Colleague 1   I heard our organisation is considering more flexible working hours next year.

Colleague 2   That's great news – a more **accommodating** / *flexible* **policy** could really help improve work-life balance for everyone.

Referral Letter / Discharge Summary

We have adjusted our treatment plan to **accommodate** / *adhere to* the patient's strong preference for non-surgical interventions.

Scientific Literature

As the infection rate rises significantly and this is followed by a dramatic increase in mortality, the whole world is struggling to **accommodate change** and is trying to adapt to new conditions. Aydogdu, M.O. et al. (2021).

However, many developing countries have fragile health systems and find it difficult to **accommodate change**. Brooks, A. et al. (2012).

[...] breeding sea cucumbers can **accommodate** the high oxygen **demand** by accelerating respiratory rate. Ru, X. et al. (2020).

acquiesce (vi) C2

Word family: adj: acquiescent; n: acquiescence ; syn: assent

to accept something without protest, despite potential personal disagreement or reservations

+ prep | in, to

Dialogue

Patient   I've been hesitant about trying this new medication.

Doctor   I understand, but if you're willing to **acquiesce** / *try it out*, we can start with a low dose and monitor how you respond.

Q&A

Questioner   Have you considered the potential long-term side effects of the new drug, particularly in patients with compromised liver function?

Presenter   We are not **acquiescent** / *willing* **to** rush the drug to market without a comprehensive long-term safety profile, especially for at-risk populations.

Informal

Colleague 1   Have you met our new colleague in the cardiology department?

Colleague 2   Yeah, she seems nice although a bit too **acquiescent** / *willing* **to** please others for my liking. It would be nice to know what she really thinks.

Referral Letter / Discharge Summary

Although initially reluctant, the patient has become more **acquiescent to** / *accepting of* the idea of cognitive behavioural therapy as a treatment option for their anxiety disorder.

Scientific Literature

Clinicians report that they routinely receive requests to delay vaccines and that they routinely **acquiesce**. Jacobson, R.M. et al. (2015).

The interviewer provided positive reinforcement when children **acquiesced to** suggestions and negative feedback when they did not. Cleveland, K.C. et al. (2016).

People can detect an error, but choose not to correct it, a process I refer to as **acquiescence**. Risen, J.L. (2016).

ENGLISH EXPRESSIONS IN CONTEXT

advocate (vt, vi, n) C1 C2

Word family: n: advocacy

to publicly endorse or recommend an idea, plan or approach; (n) a person who supports or argues in favour of someone or something

(v): + n | **policy, practice | use | view** | + prep | **for** | exp | **be widely advocated** |
adj | **leading, outspoken, prominent | ardent*** | + (n) | **of, for**

Dialogue

Patient What do you think could be causing my frequent headaches lately?

Doctor To determine the underlying cause, I'd **advocate** / *recommend* the **use** of a targeted migraine medication alongside a comprehensive neurological evaluation.

Q&A

Questioner There are different ways to approach implementation of this new treatment in clinical practice – what would you recommend?

Presenter I **advocate** the **view** / *recommend* that this treatment should be gradually introduced, starting with patients who have not responded well to conventional therapies.

Informal

Colleague 1 I heard rumours that your team is working on a new targeted therapy for pancreatic cancer – is that true?

Colleague 2 Absolutely, and while we're still in the preclinical stage, as **an advocate** / *a strong supporter* of personalised medicine, I'm really excited about its potential to improve patient outcomes.

Referral Letter / Discharge Summary

As her primary care physician, I strongly **advocate for** / *recommend* Ms. Johnson's referral to a rheumatologist to investigate her atypical symptoms.

Playing **devil's advocate** / *considering an alternative perspective*, we must consider the possibility that Ms. Thompson's symptoms may be psychosomatic.

Scientific Literature

Advance care planning **is widely advocated** to improve outcomes in end-of-life care for patients suffering from heart failure. Schichtel, M. et al. (2020).

Even **ardent advocates** of guidelines acknowledge the evidence that disseminating reviews and recommendations, by itself, fails to motivate clinicians [...]. Woolf, S.H., George, J.N. (2000).

Application in context

A **devil's advocate** *is someone who argues a contrary view they don't believe, to provoke thought or encourage discussion.*

MEDICAL EDITION

affect (vt)

Word family: n: affect (mostly in psychology – refers to the experience of mood/emotion); adj: affective (uncommon)

to impact, influence or modify someone/something, resulting in a change to their state, behaviour or characteristics

adv | directly, indirectly | adversely, negatively | significantly | positively | + n as object | ability, performance, productivity | course, development, outcome, result | health, survival, well-being

Dialogue

Patient   I twisted my ankle while playing basketball, and it really hurts.

Doctor   The sprain may **affect** / *limit* your mobility temporarily, but you should be back to normal soon.

Q&A

Questioner   How do you think your research findings will impact public health policies addressing the ongoing pandemic?

Presenter   I believe our research will significantly **affect** / *impact* public health policies, by highlighting the need for a more targeted approach.

Informal

Colleague 1   I find the new work schedule challenging – what do you think?

Colleague 2   Absolutely, it's really **affecting** / *impacting* my productivity.

Referral Letter / Discharge Summary

> Recent episodes of non-adherence have adversely **affected** / *worsened* the course of her diabetes management.

Scientific Literature

> The patterns of racial disparities in health suggest that there are multiple ways by which racism can **affect** health. Williams, D.R., Mohammed, S.A. (2009).
>
> Exercise has the potential to **positively affect** patients with osteosarcoma by improvement of function, mitigation of disability, and maintenance of independence [...]. Garcia, M.B. et al. (2020).
>
> The consequences of the Court's decision will **directly affect** the future of medicine in the United States. Cohen, J.J. (2003).
>
> PM2.5 could also **indirectly affect** the brain via activation of a localized inflammatory response in the cardiovascular system [...]. Zhang, B. et al. (2023).

Application in context

> **affect** *is usually a verb meaning 'to influence something', while* **effect** *is usually a noun meaning 'result' but can sometimes be a verb meaning 'to make happen'. See page 110.*

ENGLISH EXPRESSIONS IN CONTEXT

aggravate (vi)

Word family: n: aggravation; adj: aggravating, aggravated

to intensify or worsen an illness or negative circumstance; to irritate or provoke someone, often intentionally

+ n as object | condition, injury, symptom | situation, problem |
adv | seriously, severely | slightly

Dialogue

Patient I've been experiencing a lot of pain in my lower back lately, especially after sitting for long periods at work.

Doctor Based on your description and the physical examination, it appears that prolonged sitting is severely **aggravating** / *worsening* your lumbar spine condition.

Q&A

Questioner Regarding the potential side effects of this medication, could you elaborate on how it might affect patients with pre-existing conditions?

Presenter While this medication is generally well-tolerated, it may **aggravate** / *worsen* symptoms in patients with certain pre-existing conditions, such as hypertension or diabetes.

Informal

Colleague 1 You seemed a bit frustrated during the Q&A session earlier – is everything alright?

Colleague 2 Yeah, I was just dealing with some **aggravation** / *annoyance* from the constant interruptions and off-topic questions.

Referral Letter / Discharge Summary

Physical exertion appeared to **aggravate** / *worsen* her symptoms of lower back pain and sciatica*. The **aggravation** / *worsening* typically lasted for 2–3 hours following any prolonged standing or walking.

Scientific Literature

Despite their clinical relevance, there is a surprisingly limited availability of clinically approved antifungal agents, which is **seriously aggravated** by the recent appearance and fast spread of drug resistance. Amich, J. (2022).

In patients with ischemic heart disease, myocardial ischemia-reperfusion injury (IRI) can **aggravate** their **condition** even worse [...]. Tian, H. et al. (2021).

Subsequent revisionary procedures not only failed to reduce the tip size but **aggravated** the **problem** causing an even larger and less defined nasal tip. Gruber, R.P. et al. (2018).

MEDICAL EDITION

aggregate (vt) `C1` `C2`

Word family: n: aggregation

(usually passive) to combine items or amounts into a single total; (adj) made up of several amounts added together; (n) a total formed by combining smaller quantities

vt + n as object | **information, data** |
adj + n | **effect** | **amount, value** | **output, score**

Dialogue

Patient What is causing my persistent headaches and fatigue?

Doctor I'll need to **aggregate** / *collect* **information** from various tests to determine the underlying cause of your symptoms.

Q&A

Questioner Could you elaborate on how the combined treatments affected patient outcomes?

Presenter Our research demonstrated a significant **aggregate** / *overall* **effect** of these interventions, leading to improved long-term prognoses.

Informal

Colleague 1 How's your team's productivity been this quarter?

Colleague 2 Pretty good – thanks to the new workflow system, our **aggregate** / *overall* **output** has increased substantially.

Referral Letter / Discharge Summary

After careful **aggregation** / *compilation* of the patient's lab results, imaging studies and clinical presentation, we recommend a multidisciplinary approach for this complex case.

Scientific Literature

Some, but not all, strains of Streptococcus sanguis have been reported to **aggregate** platelets but [...]. Douglas, C.W. et al. (1990).

Both **aggregate** and individual analyses are valid, although they provide answers to different questions. O'Leary, K.D., Woodin, E.M. (2005).

This phenomenon is considered based on a model system as wetting of a cell **aggregate** on a rigid substrate [...]. Pajic-Lijakovic, I., Milivojevic, M. (2023).

ENGLISH EXPRESSIONS IN CONTEXT

anecdotal (adj)

Word family: n: anecdote; adv: anecdotally

(of a report or evidence) based on personal stories rather than verified facts or scientific research, potentially reducing reliability or accuracy

+ n | evidence, information, report

Dialogue

Patient   Is acupuncture something you would recommend for my condition?

Doctor   While there have been some **anecdotal reports** / *stories* of improvement, I suggest that we pursue a treatment plan backed by scientific evidence.

Q&A

Questioner   You mentioned that some patients reported improvements with the treatment, but how strong is the data supporting those claims?

Presenter   While we've observed promising results, much of what I shared today relies on **anecdotal evidence** / *personal experiences* from individual cases.

Informal

Colleague 1   Did you hear about that new restaurant that opened down the street?

Colleague 2   Yes, I heard some **anecdotal stories** / *people's opinions* about it, but I haven't had a chance to try it yet.

Referral Letter / Discharge Summary

The patient's history of migraine triggers remains largely based on **anecdotal information** / *personal accounts* from family members, as she has been unable to maintain a consistent headache diary due to cognitive difficulties.

Scientific Literature

So far, few mechanism-based treatments for phantom-limb pain have been proposed. Most published reports are based on **anecdotal evidence**. Flor, H. (2002).

Recent evidence, as well as **anecdotal information**, suggests that athletes may experience a reduced quality and/or quantity of sleep. Halson, S.L. (2014).

Often the decisions made by clinicians are made from **anecdotes** or guidelines that may be out of date or supported by low-quality evidence. Mohajir, W.A. et al. (2022).

The presence of dengue virus in – and human-to-human, non-vector transmission from – various bodily fluids other than semen or vaginal secretions has been documented **anecdotally**. Several **anecdotal reports** described prolonged presence of DENV (dengue virus) in semen, urine and vaginal secretions. Grobusch, M.P. et al. (2020).

anomaly (n) C1 C2

Word family: adj: anomalous

something that deviates from what is usual or anticipated

adj + | congenital

Dialogue

Patient My stomach has been hurting terribly for weeks, and now I feel a hard lump just above my right hip.

Doctor The X-ray reveals an **anomaly** / *abnormality* in your lower intestine that requires immediate surgery.

Q&A

Questioner How do you explain the **anomaly** / *discrepancy* (or inconsistency) in your data showing a lower remission rate compared to those from previous studies?

Presenter I believe our larger sample size provides a more accurate representation of real-world outcomes.

Informal

Colleague 1 That **anomaly** / *unexpected issue* in the scheduling system had me double-booked for procedures all afternoon.

Colleague 2 I dealt with that last week – I had patients showing up who weren't even on my list.

Referral Letter / Discharge Summary

Upon chest X-ray imaging performed on 12/14/2024, a small **anomaly** / *abnormality* was detected in the right lower lobe, necessitating further investigation with contrast-enhanced CT scanning.

Scientific Literature

Up to 90% of infants with an **anomaly** involving the left coronary artery die within the first year of life if left untreated. Goo, H.W. (2021).

We discuss 6 of the more common **anomalous** muscles encountered by hand surgeons [...]. Andring, N. et al. (2018).

The prevalence of **congenital anomalies** in Europe (article title). Dolk, H. et al. (2010).

Ebstein **anomaly** is a congenital malformation involving primarily the tricuspid valve, with failure of delamination from the underlying myocardium and right ventricular myopathy. Fuchs, M.M., Connolly, H.M. (2020).

ENGLISH EXPRESSIONS IN CONTEXT

appraise (vt) `C1`

Word family: n: appraisal

to assess or evaluate a person or thing by examining them/it carefully and forming a judgment

---

+ n as object | **situation** | **quality** | + prep | **of**

Dialogue

Patient My stomach has been hurting for days.

Doctor I'll need to **appraise** / *assess* the situation before making any recommendations.

Q&A

Questioner How did you **appraise** / *evaluate* the efficacy of the new treatment protocol in your study?

Presenter We used a combination of patient-reported outcomes and clinical assessments over a six-month period.

Informal

Colleague 1 Have you seen the new art exhibition at the city museum?

Colleague 2 Not yet, but I'm planning to go this weekend to **appraise** / *check out* the collection. I'll let you know if it's worth it.

Referral Letter / Discharge Summary

> I am referring Mrs. Anderson to your care so that we may jointly **appraise** / *evaluate* the **situation** regarding her persistent abdominal pain, which has not responded to conventional treatments.

Scientific Literature

> Generally, assessing random and systematic errors is necessary to **appraise** study **quality** rather than relying on ambiguous labels. Korsgaard, S., Schmidt, M. (2024).
>
> Stress includes not only the stimulus and the response but also the individual **appraisal of** the **situation**. Koolhaas, J.M. et al. (2016).
>
> It is necessary to evaluate single positivities and negativities, but also to **appraise** "the big picture" with perspective. Luengo, O., Cardona, V. (2014).

MEDICAL EDITION

attenuate (vt)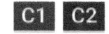

Word family: n: attenuation; adj: attenuated

to reduce the strength or effectiveness of something

adv | **effectively** | **gradually**

Dialogue

Patient The pain feels like a hot poker* stabbing me in the back and keeps me awake all night.

Doctor We can **attenuate** / *reduce* your discomfort with a combination of physical therapy and anti-inflammatory medication.

Q&A

Questioner How did your treatment affect the inflammatory markers in rheumatoid arthritis patients?

Presenter Our treatment **attenuated** / *reduced* IL-6 levels by up to 40% within the first month.

Informal

Colleague 1 The new coffee machine in the break room makes the worst coffee I've ever tasted.

Colleague 2 This charcoal filter should significantly **attenuate** / *reduce* (or *decrease, lessen*) the bitter, burnt flavour everyone's been complaining about.

Referral Letter / Discharge Summary

The patient responded well to methotrexate, which helped **attenuate** / *reduce* her joint inflammation and morning stiffness. **Gradual attenuation** / *reduction* of symptoms over six weeks allowed her to resume normal daily activities.

Scientific Literature

Platelet-rich plasma has been widely popular in facial rejuvenation to **attenuate** wrinkles and has been practically used. Uysal, C.A., Ertas, N.M. (2017).

Systemic glucocorticoid therapy may **effectively attenuate** lung inflammation but also induce severe side-effects. Hegeman, M.A. et al. (2011).

Resistance exercise training induces skeletal muscle hypertrophy, but repeated bouts **gradually attenuate** this anabolic effect. Takegaki, J. et al. (2019).

ENGLISH EXPRESSIONS IN CONTEXT

battered (adj)

Word family: vi/vt: batter (= to hit somebody/something hard many times, especially in a way that causes serious damage)

worn, heavily used and deteriorated; physically harmed through repeated violent assault; severely damaged by weaponry or harsh environmental conditions

v + | be, feel, look | become | + n | child, woman | exp | battered and bruised

Dialogue

Doctor   How have you been feeling since your accident last week?

Patient   To be honest, I **feel** completely **battered** / *broken*, both physically and emotionally, and I'm struggling to cope with the pain and anxiety.

Q&A

Questioner   Could you elaborate on how the long-term stress on the body might manifest in patients?

Presenter   When patients are subjected to chronic stress, their physical and mental well-being can **become battered** / *severely impacted* over time, leading to a host of health issues.

Informal

Colleague 1   I heard you've been working on the project non-stop lately – honestly, you look **battered** / *exhausted*.

Colleague 2   Yeah, but I'm making good progress, and the results are promising. I just need to push through this final stretch.

Referral Letter / Discharge Summary

> The patient's presentation was consistent with **Battered** / (*abused*) Woman Syndrome, prompting immediate referral to our hospital's domestic violence support services and social work team.

Scientific Literature

> **Battered Child** Syndrome seems to be a relatively common phenomenon, as a great majority of participants (86.25%) had encountered it in their practice. Pabis, M. et al. (2011).
>
> A recent study in a large metropolitan area documented one in twelve pregnant women to have been physically **battered** during the present pregnancy. McFarlane, J. (1989).
>
> Our approach to measuring **battering** operationalizes the experiences of **battered women** rather than the abusive behaviours they encounter. Smith, P.H. et al. (1995).

Application in context

> *Battered Person Syndrome is a psychological condition resulting from prolonged abuse. Although recognised in medical and legal fields, it is not classified in DSM-5.*

MEDICAL EDITION

benevolent (adj) C2

Word family: n: benevolence*;
adv: benevolently; ant: malevolent

showing kindness and generosity; donating money or support to those in need or to charitable organisations

+ n | society | fund, funding | leadership | work

Dialogue

Patient   I've been putting off coming in because I don't have insurance.

Doctor   We have a **benevolent** / *charitable* fund that can help cover your treatment costs if needed.

Q&A

Questioner   Your results seem to suggest a **benevolent** / *favourable* prognosis for most patients, but I wonder if you've considered age-related comorbidities?

Presenter   Yes, we stratified patients by age and adjusted for major comorbidities in our analysis.

Informal

Colleague 1   I'm thinking of switching my research focus to pediatric neuroplasticity next year.

Colleague 2   That would be a **benevolent** / *worthwhile* cause, with good funding opportunities.

Referral Letter / Discharge Summary

Despite the patient's financial hardship, she was able to receive full treatment through hospital **benevolence funding** / *charitable assistance*.

Scientific Literature

Thomas Hodgkin was a diligent, selfless and **benevolent** man whose name is instantly recognisable in the medical field due to his description of a type of the lymphoma that is named after him, 'Hodgkin's Lymphoma'. Wells, E. (2017).

The results showed that work engagement mediated **benevolent leadership** and job performance. Lee, M.C.C., Ding, A.Y.L. (2024).

Consent for organ donation in a brain dead patient represents an act of **benevolence** or of solidarity in favour of an unknown person. Beloucif, S. (2012).

Throughout the interaction, a receiver is matched with the same sender who is either malevolent with an objective opposed to the receiver or **benevolent** always telling the truth. Ettinger, D., Jehiel, P. (2021).

ENGLISH EXPRESSIONS IN CONTEXT

bolster (vt)

Word family: n: bolster

to strengthen or enhance something, providing support or reinforcement

+ n as object |argument, case, claim, theory | confidence, support | morale | reputation

Dialogue

Patient My shoulder hurts whenever I raise my arm above my head.

Doctor I'll prescribe physical therapy exercises to **bolster** / *strengthen* your rotator cuff muscles.

Q&A

Questioner How did your novel treatment impact patient-compliance rates?

Presenter Our data shows that weekly text message reminders **bolster** / *increase* patient adherence by 30%.

Informal

Colleague 1 After three failed grant applications, I'm really doubting my research capabilities.

Colleague 2 Let me take you out for coffee and **bolster** / *lift* your morale with some stories about my own early rejections that led to better opportunities.

Referral Letter / Discharge Summary

The patient reports seeking a second opinion from our university medical center to **bolster** / *validate* our **reputation** for expertise in rare autoimmune conditions, but our findings align with those of her local rheumatologist.

Scientific Literature

These findings **bolster** the **argument** for routine cholangiography as a safe, effective, and helpful screening examination for patients who are at risk for having common bile duct disease. Shively, E.H. et al. (1990).

Clinical research incorporating standardised hypothetical decision-making protocols, as well as triangulated data collection methods, would **bolster confidence** in future findings. Spalding, R. (2021).

The postpandemic atmosphere has created a perfect storm that has necessitated a renewed prioritization to **bolster support** for the role of the clinical nurse manager. Buck, C.K. et al (2023).

circumvent (vt) C2

Word family: n: circumvention

to cleverly or strategically bypass an obstacle, rule or restriction by finding an alternative path or method around it

+ n as object | limitation | danger, difficulty, issue, obstacle, problem | challenge | rule, law | need

Dialogue

Patient   My shoulder has been killing me lately when I lift weights.

Doctor   To **circumvent** / *avoid* the **risk** of permanent injury, I'd recommend taking a two-week break from all upper-body exercises and applying ice three times daily.

Q&A

Questioner   Have you considered how reduced blood flow might affect your proposed treatment method?

Presenter   We were able to **circumvent** / *overcome* that **obstacle** by incorporating a vasodilator into the protocol.

Informal

Colleague 1   Our new department chair seems really strict about everyone taking their full lunch hour.

Colleague 2   I know, but I have so much work! I **circumvent** / *get around* that rule by eating at my desk while catching up on research papers.

Referral Letter / Discharge Summary

> To **circumvent** / *overcome* the **challenge** of her medication intolerance, we initiated a gradual desensitisation protocol under close monitoring.

Scientific Literature

> Careful and diligent management of tracheostomy patients can **circumvent** many **problems** and allow the patient to breath with less difficulty. Hedlund, C.S. (1991).

> Regarding the increasing prevalence of cancer throughout the globe, the development of novel alternatives for conventional therapies is inevitable to **circumvent limitations** such as low efficacy, complications, and high cost. Alimardani, V. (2021).

> In contrast, novel learning rules based on the information bottleneck (IB) train each layer of a network independently, **circumventing** the **need** to propagate errors across layers. Daruwalla, K., Lipasti, M. (2024).

ENGLISH EXPRESSIONS IN CONTEXT

cognitive (adj) C1

Word family: n: cognition; syn: mental

related to mental processes involved in understanding and thinking

+ n | bias | development | ability, disability | function | process | psychology, neuroscience, science | skill | theory | therapy

Dialogue

Patient I keep forgetting where I put my keys and other important things lately.

Doctor Based on your symptoms and test results, I believe you're experiencing early signs of **cognitive** / *mental* **decline**.

Q&A

Questioner How was sleep deprivation related to **cognitive** / *mental* **skills** in your study?

Presenter Contrary to our expectations, we did not find any relationship between the two.

Informal

Colleague 1 Did you catch that fascinating documentary last night about how video games might actually enhance brain function in older adults?

Colleague 2 Yes, and I was particularly struck by how the **cognitive** / *mental* **benefits** lasted even months after they stopped playing.

Referral Letter / Discharge Summary

Ms. T demonstrates intact **cognitive processes** / *mental functioning* across all domains, with particularly strong performance in memory, attention and executive function tasks during her neuropsychological assessment. Her overall **cognition** / *mental* **capacity** appears to be age-appropriate with no indication of decline over the past year.

Scientific Literature

Sleep is important for brain health, having both a restorative function and playing an important role in **cognitive functions**, e.g., attention, memory, learning, and planning. Amidi, A. et al. (2023).

A **cognitive bias** describes "shortcuts" subconsciously applied to new scenarios to simplify decision-making. Richburg, C.E. et al. (2023).

Over a century of psychological research provides strong and consistent support for the idea that **cognitive ability** correlates positively with success in tasks that people face in employment, education, and everyday life. Beier, M.E., Oswald, F.L. (2012).

MEDICAL EDITION

compensate (vi)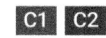

Word family: n: compensation adj: compensable

to offset harm or loss by providing something beneficial; to correct an imbalance or deficiency; to reimburse someone for damage, loss or injury

+ n as object | victim | workers

Dialogue

Patient   My knee has been giving me terrible pain lately, especially when I climb stairs.

Doctor   Don't worry – your other leg will naturally **compensate** / *take over* while this one heals.

Q&A

Questioner   Could you explain how your data accounts for the wide age range of your study participants?

Presenter   We **compensate** / *adjust* **for** the age variability by normalising each result against the participant's baseline measurements.

Informal

Colleague 1   I'm worried that this morning's surgery might be delayed because of the power cuts we've been experiencing lately.

Colleague 2   Don't worry – backup generators have been installed to **compensate** / *make up* **for** that, just in case.

Referral Letter / Discharge Summary

> The patient's right kidney appears to **compensate** / *make up* **for** the reduced function of the left kidney. This renal **compensation** / *adjustment* is evidenced by the increased size and filtration rate of the right kidney noted on imaging studies.

Scientific Literature

> In many cases an on-road driving test to evaluate the ability to **compensate for** functional impairments is essential. Brunnauer, A. et al. (2014).
>
> The primary goal of the Dutch Institute for Asbestos Victims is to **compensate** mesothelioma victims who have been exposed to asbestos in the workplace [...]. Waterman, Y.R., Peeters, M.G. (2004).
>
> [...] the authors present a comparative analysis of the law of medical negligence in this context and a discussion of the grounds for **compensable** injury resulting from medical error Scurria, S. et al. (2019).

ENGLISH EXPRESSIONS IN CONTEXT

compound (vt)

Word family: adj: compunding; syn: worsen

to intensify or escalate an already negative situation by adding further difficulties or harm

+ n as object | difficulty, issue, problem, situation | effect | stress | risk

Dialogue

Patient   I've been feeling so overwhelmed lately – between the chronic pain and the stress at work, it's hard to manage.

Doctor   I understand. Chronic pain can often **compound** / *add to* **difficulties** like stress and fatigue. Let's work on a plan to address both issues together.

Q&A

Questioner   How might the simultaneous use of multiple medications **compound** / *increase* health **risks** for elderly patients?

Presenter   Polypharmacy* in geriatric populations significantly increases the likelihood of drug-drug interactions and related complications.

Informal

Colleague 1   I heard the project deadline got moved up by two weeks.

Colleague 2   Yeah, and to **compound** the **problem** / *make matters worse*, our lead researcher just called in sick for the rest of the week.

Referral Letter / Discharge Summary

The patient's chronic pain appears to **compound** / *worsen* the **stress** from her recent job loss, potentially exacerbating her depressive symptoms.

Scientific Literature

The COVID pandemic seems to have further **compounded** the **problem** and the possibility of 'missed' or 'delayed' diagnosis is ever-present. Paling, C. (2021).

Serum levels of vitamins A and E **compounded** the **effect** of low selenium [...]. Willet, W.C. et al. (1983).

Tobacco use was found to **compound risks** associated with diabetes (n = 1), cancer (n = 2), and chronic liver disease (n = 1). Baker, J. et al. (2022).

MEDICAL EDITION

concede (vt, vi) C1 C2

Word family: n: concession; syn: admit

(vt) to acknowledge truth after initially denying it; (vi/vt) to recognise one's loss in a contest or election; to reluctantly surrender or yield something

+ n as object | point | possibility | defeat | election |
v + | be forced to | be prepared to

Dialogue

Patient My back pain hasn't improved despite following your treatment plan for a month.

Doctor I must **concede** / *admit* that your case is more complex than I initially thought.

Q&A

Questioner While I **concede** that / *Even though* vaccines have been effective against many diseases, aren't there still risks associated with their use?

Presenter Research consistently shows that vaccines provide substantial protection against deadly diseases, with serious side effects being extremely rare.

Informal

Colleague 1 Don't you think it would be better for everyone's health if we replaced the vending machine with a healthier snack bar in the break room?

Colleague 2 I **concede** / *admit* that **point**, but we might face some pushback from staff who enjoy an occasional treat after a hard day's work.

Referral Letter / Discharge Summary

Even the most experienced specialists **were forced to concede** / *accept* (or *admit*) that Mr. Johnson's symptoms did not fit any typical pattern of autoimmune disease. This **concession** / *acknowledgement* led to a broader investigative approach, ultimately revealing a rare genetic disorder that explained his constellation of symptoms.

Scientific Literature

In our opinion, it is not sufficient for the tobacco industry to merely **concede** the obvious **point** that smoking is a cause of disease [...]. Cummings, K,M, et al, (2007).

The majority of respondents (n = 22, 66.7%) **conceded** the **possibility** of identifier-contained unstructured data in the NOTE table. Tak, Y.W. et al. (2022).

However, doing so would require **making concessions** they would be unlikely to make, the crucial one being subscribing to an absurd view that [...]. Dominiak, Ł. (2024).

ENGLISH EXPRESSIONS IN CONTEXT

concurrent (adj) C1

Word family: adv: concurrently; n: concurrency

occurring, existing or operating simultaneously; taking place during the same timeframe

+ n as object | use | + prep | with

Dialogue

Patient My migraines haven't improved despite taking the prescribed medication daily.

Doctor There may be a **concurrent** / *coexisting* hormonal imbalance contributing to your symptoms, which we'll need to investigate further.

Q&A

Questioner Could you elaborate on your analysis of drug interactions in elderly patients taking both statins and beta blockers?

Presenter Our data showed that **concurrent** / *simultaneous* use of these medications increased fall risk in patients over 75 years old.

Informal

Colleague 1 The **concurrent** / *parallel* development of AI diagnostics and robotic surgery is revolutionising modern medicine.

Colleague 2 Yes, and I'm particularly excited about how this combination is reducing recovery times for patients.

Referral Letter / Discharge Summary

The patient is being treated with metformin for type 2 diabetes and is **concurrently** / *simultaneously* receiving chemotherapy for stage 2 breast cancer.

Scientific Literature

Fifty-four psychiatric inpatients identified by hospital staff as having delusions were interviewed about their history of delusions and incidents of violence that were **concurrent with** delusions. Junginger, J. et al. (1998).

Concurrent use of cannabis and alcohol is frequent. Romaguera, A. et al. (2017).

We examined the predictors of excess body weight (EBW) **concurrently** affecting mother-child pairs after delivery during 6 years of follow-up. Czarnobay, S.A. et al. (2023).

Application in context

*concurrent vs. simultaneous: in medical contexts, **concurrent** describes overlapping conditions or treatments, while **simultaneous** refers to events occurring at exactly the same moment.*

MEDICAL EDITION

conducive (adj)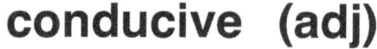

Word family: n: conduciveness

creating favourable conditions for something to occur or making it more likely to happen

+ n as object or subject | **environment, atmosphere** |
adv + | **highly** | **especially** | + prep | **to**

Dialogue

Doctor How have you been feeling since our last appointment?

Patient Well, I've tried to create an atmosphere more **conducive to** / *better for* relaxation – it seems to help with my stress levels.

Q&A

Questioner Have you considered investigating whether certain environmental factors are **conducive to** / *helpful for* the observed outcomes in your study?

Presenter While I didn't explicitly mention it, we are currently exploring the impact of certain environmental factors.

Informal

Colleague 1 How's your new job treating you?

Colleague 2 I am lucky to be in an **environment conducive to** / *good place for* continuing my research.

Referral Letter / Discharge Summary

> Environmental factors at home, including a recently installed air purifier and hypoallergenic bedding, seem **conducive to** / *appear helpful for* (or *look suitable for*) managing the patient's chronic asthma symptoms more effectively.

Scientific Literature

> [...] it is essential that students learn medicine in a **conducive environment** of public hospitals, community clinics and health posts. Vento, S. (2023).
>
> Bivariate analysis shows that **conducive atmosphere** at workplace, favourable attitude of colleagues and husband/in-laws, and sharing their own problems with husband have significant positive impact on mental health outcomes of married working women. Panigrahi, A. et al. (2014).
>
> However, results also draw attention to the critical role of economic, social, and healthcare policies for creating an **environment** that is **conducive to** following medical recommendations. Oates, G.R. et al. (2020).

ENGLISH EXPRESSIONS IN CONTEXT

confer (vt, vi)

Word family: n: conference

to discuss issues with others for opinions or advice; (vt) to grant honours, degrees or rights; to transmit qualities or characteristics to something

+ n as object | **resistance, tolerance** | **protection** | **risk**

Dialogue

Patient Why do I seem to catch every cold that goes around the office?

Doctor A deficiency in vitamin D can **confer** / *lead to* increased **susceptibility** to respiratory infections.

Q&A

Questioner Could you explain why some patients still develop thrombosis despite taking aspirin?

Presenter Our research shows that certain genetic variants can **confer** / *lead to* **resistance** to antiplatelet therapy, including aspirin.

Informal

Colleague 1 It's fascinating how some bilingual people I know never seem to develop dementia, even well into their 80s.

Colleague 2 Yes, speaking multiple languages appears to **confer** / *provide* significant **protection** against cognitive decline in ageing.

Referral Letter / Discharge Summary

> Given the risk profile of this patient, coexisting type 2 diabetes and chronic kidney disease **confer** / *create* a significantly elevated **risk** of cardiovascular complications in the post-operative period.

Scientific Literature

> Members of the ATP-binding cassette F (ABC-F) proteins **confer resistance** to several classes of clinically important antibiotics through ribosome protection. Ero, R. et al. (2019).
>
> Thus, a successful Zika vaccine needs to not only **confer protection** from ZIKV infection but must also be safe during secondary exposures with other flavivirus [...]. Wang, R. et al. (2019).
>
> These cells **confer** multi-drug **tolerance**, to targeted and chemotherapies alike, until the residual disease can establish a stable, drug-resistant state. Moore, P.C. et al. (2023).

Application in context

*The second meaning of **confer** ('to transmit qualities or characteristics to something') is commonly used in scientific contexts, extending the meaning 'to give or grant' to describe properties, characteristics or effects rather than awards or honours.*

MEDICAL EDITION

congruent (adj)

Word family: n: congruence/congruency; adv: congruently; ant: incongruent; syn: compatible

harmoniously aligned, matching or compatible with something else, allowing both to exist together without conflict or contradiction

+ prep | **with, to** | + n as object | **number**

Dialogue

Patient My right knee hurts whenever I bend it to climb stairs.

Doctor Your symptoms appear **congruent with** / *match* early onset osteoarthritis.

Q&A

Questioner How do your findings relate to Smith's study from last year?

Presenter Our results are **congruent** / *align* **with** Smith's, though we examined a larger patient cohort.

Informal

Colleague 1 Did the lab results come back yet?

Colleague 2 Yeah, they're **congruent** / *match* **with** what we were expecting. No surprises.

Referral Letter / Discharge Summary

> The patient's physical exam findings show **congruency with** / *agree with* the radiological studies, confirming right hip osteoarthritis.

Scientific Literature

> Recent behavioral studies have shown that color imagery can benefit visual search when it is **congruent with** an upcoming target. Cochrane, B.A. et al. (2021).
>
> The appropriate interpretation of the target was either **congruent** or **incongruent with** the cue presented in a subsequent word association task. Zeelenberg, R. et al. (2003).
>
> The role of parental **congruence** in pre-school children's screen time, moderated by parental education (article title). Burnett, A.J. et al. (2023).
>
> We found that infants were able to discriminate **congruently** (same direction) vs. **incongruently** moving (opposite direction) pairs irrespective of modality (Experiment 1). Nava, E. et al. (2017).

ENGLISH EXPRESSIONS IN CONTEXT

conjure (vt, vi) `C1`

Word family: n: conjuration

to perform skilful tricks that make objects seem to appear or vanish, as if by magic

+ n as object | **image, memory, mental image** |
phrV | **conjure up**

Dialogue

Patient I've been really forgetful lately, and it's concerning me.

Doctor It's common to forget things as we age, but there are techniques we can explore to help **conjure up** / *bring back* those **memories**.

Q&A

Questioner How did you manage to come up with the surgical approach for this case so quickly and efficiently?

Presenter We carefully considered the patient's condition and medical history to **conjure up** / *figure out* the most appropriate surgical strategy.

Informal

Colleague 1 How's your day going so far? Are you enjoying the conference?

Colleague 2 It's been great – the presentations have been fascinating, and they've **conjured up** / *sparked* some exciting new ideas for my research.

Referral Letter / Discharge Summary

The patient describes a tendency for certain triggers to **conjure** / *form* vivid and intrusive **mental images**, often tied to past traumatic events. These episodes are accompanied by significant emotional distress and impact their daily functioning.

Scientific Literature

With effort, most literate persons can **conjure** more or less vague visual **mental images** of the written form of words they are hearing [...]. Hauw, F. et al. (2023).

A diagnosis of cancer can **conjure up** a whole host of emotions. Reynolds, D. (2006).

Middle class, middle aged, female: I can hear the yawns already. This is not a description to **conjure up** the **image** of a forward-thinking, hard-working dentist with a wide portfolio outside her chosen profession. Wiles, L. (1991).

MEDICAL EDITION

consistent (adj)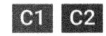

Word family: n: consistency; adv: consistently; ant: inconsistent

behaving or thinking steadily with unchanged standards; occurring uniformly over time; consistent/agreeing with something; having logically aligned ideas or arguments

v | be | + prep | across, among | with | adv | internally, logically

Dialogue

Patient   I've been experiencing headaches lately.

Doctor   Have these headaches **been consistent** / *similar* in terms of intensity?

Q&A

Questioner   How **consistent** / *similar* **were** the experimental results across different trial runs?

Presenter   The experimental results exhibited remarkable **consistency** / *stayed nearly the same* throughout various trial runs.

Informal

Colleague 1   Was the conference content **consistent** / *aligned* **with** what you were hoping to learn?

Colleague 2   Definitely, the topics aligned perfectly with my expectations.

Referral Letter / Discharge Summary

The patient's elevated blood pressure readings **were consistent** / *remained the same* **across** multiple clinic visits over the past three months.

Scientific Literature

These results are **consistent with** observations of night migratory behaviour in animals at low light levels and [...]. Zoltowski, B.D. et al. (2019).

[...] informant reports tended to be more **internally consistent** than self reports, as indicated by equal or higher Cronbach's alpha scores and higher average interitem correlations. Balsis, S. et al. (2015).

All region-specific results **consistently** suggested a link between PM2·5 and first Parkinson's disease and Alzheimer's disease and related dementias hospital admissions, although effect estimates varied by geographical region. Shi, L. et al. (2020).

Application in context

*consistent vs. constant: both terms imply steadiness, but **consistent** refers to maintaining reliability or quality over time, even with intervals, while **constant** denotes something continuous and uninterrupted.*

ENGLISH EXPRESSIONS IN CONTEXT

consolidate (vt, vi)

Word family: n: consolidation

to strengthen and secure power or success for lasting stability; to combine multiple elements into a single, unified whole

+ n as object | **debt, gain | data | progress**

Dialogue

Patient   I've been feeling better lately, but I'm worried that the progress won't last.

Doctor   You've made great strides. Now, we'll focus on **consolidating** / *adding to* your **progress** to ensure your recovery is long-term.

Q&A

Questioner   How will you address the disparate data sources in multi-centre clinical trials?

Presenter   Our team plans to **consolidate** / *integrate* the **data** from various institutions into a centralised, standardised database for more efficient analysis.

Informal

Colleague 1   It would really be worth sharing what we learned from the talks with our colleagues.

Colleague 2   I will **consolidate** / *gather* the main points from all the talks I attended into a summary report for our team.

Referral Letter / Discharge Summary

We recommend that Dr. Johnson **consolidates** / *combines* the patient's multiple prescriptions to reduce potential drug interactions and improve adherence.

Scientific Literature

[...] sleep constitutes an optimal state for the brain to reprocess and **consolidate** previous experiences. Staresina, B.P. (2024).

The guidelines **consolidate** more than 20 sets of WHO recommendations and good practice statements in one user-friendly format. No authors listed (2019).

Debt consolidation* and credit counselling will be appropriate for many individuals who have compulsive buying disorder. Black, D.W. (2001).

MEDICAL EDITION

contradict (vt, vi) [C1]

Word family: n: contradiction; adj: contradictory

(of people) to state the opposite of another's claim; (of facts/statements) to be so inconsistent with each other that one must be false

+ n as object | **belief, expectation, theory** | **finding** | **view** |
+ n as subject | **evidence, finding**

Dialogue

Patient   I've been feeling perfectly fine lately, doctor.

Doctor   The MRI findings **contradict** / *disagree with* your reported lack of **symptoms**.

Q&A

Questioner   Your study results **contradicted** / *challenged* our **expectations** regarding treatment efficacy in elderly patients.

Presenter   We were equally surprised by the outcomes, which underscore the need for age-specific clinical trials in this population.

Informal

Colleague 1   The latest findings on gut microbiome and mental health seem quite **contradictory** / *opposite* to previous research.

Colleague 2   The upcoming meta-analysis should help clarify these disparate results.

Referral Letter / Discharge Summary

> The patient's rapid improvement **contradicts** / *challenges* our initial **belief** about the severity of the condition.

Scientific Literature

> Although these approaches **contradict** each other, each of them has their own substantiating advantages and disadvantages in medical practice. Mandal, J. et al. (2016).
>
> However, findings obtained from electrophysiological and functional imaging studies over the last few years, **contradict** this **view** […]. van Luijtelaar, G. et al. (2014).
>
> Recent research has presented findings that **contradict** some of the accepted **theories** regarding the pathophysiology of some symptoms of the syndrome. Wiseman, K.C. (1991).
>
> Despite the apparent **contradiction** in the definitions of "nasal" and "local," we offer insights based on our extensive experience in the field. Bellussi, L.M. et al. (2023).

ENGLISH EXPRESSIONS IN CONTEXT

contravene (vt)

Word family: contravention; adj: contravened; syn: infringe

to breach, violate or act against an established law, regulation or official directive

+ n as object | law, regulation, rule, act, guidelines | adv | clearly, directly

Dialogue

Patient — After the surgery, I've been experiencing some unusual back pain.

Doctor — Your symptoms do raise some concerns, as they appear to **contravene** / *go against* the clear progression we were expecting.

Q&A

Questioner — In my experience, informed consent processes aren't always comprehensive, potentially putting patients at risk and challenging ethical standards.

Presenter — Our discussion highlights the potential **contraventions** / *violations* of established medical-ethics **guidelines** in certain clinical scenarios.

Informal

Colleague 1 — I noticed the new protocol for patient data sharing – did you review it?

Colleague 2 — Yes, but I'm concerned that it might **contravene** / *go against* GDPR* **guidelines** if we're not careful about obtaining explicit consent.

Note

The verb '**contravene**' appears in medical documentation discussing policy or protocol violations, or in medical ethics literature. However, it is unlikely to appear in a patient referral letter or discharge summary.

Scientific Literature

Regarding all other medications, our review found no evidence to **contravene** their use in normal therapeutic doses to G6PD-deficient patients. Youngster, I. et al. (2010).

Punishment for **contravention** of provisions of the **Act** or **rules** or **regulations** made thereunder is clear and stringent and may vary from fine to imprisonment. Chandrashekar, H. et al. (2019).

Although these experiments **contravene** widely accepted informed consent requirements and involve deception, we argue that they can be conducted ethically if risks are minimized […]. Resnik, D.B., Finn, P.R. (2018).

Application in context

contravene vs. contradict vs. controvert: **contravene** *is primarily used for violations of laws or rules, while* **contradict** *is common in general contexts to express opposition, and* **controvert** *is a formal term used in academic or legal disputes. See page* **110**.

corroborate (vt) [C2]

Word family: n: corroboration; adj: corroborative; syn: confirm

to confirm or strengthen a statement or theory with supporting evidence or information

+ n as object or subject | **finding(s), result(s)** | **theory** | **view** | **report**

Dialogue

Patient I've been noticing a persistent cough and shortness of breath, especially when I exert myself.

Doctor Your symptoms **corroborate** / *confirm* our **findings** from the chest X-ray, which show signs of chronic obstructive pulmonary disease.

Q&A

Questioner How does your research **corroborate** / *support* the **report** by Johnson on the efficacy of this new treatment in reducing inflammation markers?

Presenter Our findings show a similar reduction in inflammatory cytokines, particularly IL-6 and TNF-alpha, which aligns closely with the results presented in Johnson's paper.

Informal

Colleague 1 Hey, did you hear about Dr. Lee's latest study on the potential link between gut microbiome and Alzheimer's?

Colleague 2 Yeah, I just read it, and it's fascinating how their findings seem to **corroborate** / *confirm* some of the **theories** we've been discussing in our lab meetings about inflammation pathways.

Referral Letter / Discharge Summary

Further **corroboration** / *confirmation* of the suspected diagnosis was obtained through genetic testing, which revealed the presence of the BRCA1 mutation.

Scientific Literature

Our review of research **corroborates** the **view** that relationships are a keystone component of human functioning that have the potential to influence a broad array of mental health outcomes. Braithwaite, S., Holt-Lunstad, J. (2017).

Enzyme activity assay methods can be used to **corroborate** the **results** generated by difference gel electrophoresis (DIGE) proteomic experiments. Dowd, A. (2023).

These **findings corroborate** the latest guidelines on exercise for individuals with overweight/obesity highlighting the importance of a multicomponent exercise approach to improve cardiometabolic health. Batrakoulis, A. et al. (2022).

credible (adj) `C1`

Word family: n: credibility; adv: credibly; ant: implausible; syn: plausible, believable

worthy of acceptance or confidence; sufficiently reliable or plausible to merit trust

+ n | argument | evidence | explanation, information

Dialogue

Patient   I didn't follow the diet plan because I figured a few indulgences wouldn't hurt.

Doctor   I understand, but that's not a **credible argument** / *valid excuse*. Sticking to the plan consistently is crucial for managing your condition effectively.

Q&A

Questioner   How can your study's findings **have credibility** / *be trustworthy* with such a small sample size?

Presenter   Our rigorous methodology and statistical analysis compensate for the limited sample, yielding reliable results.

Informal

Colleague 1   Why is the project budget suddenly so much higher than we initially estimated?

Colleague 2   I don't have a **credible** / *reliable* **explanation** for the increase, but I'm investigating it right now.

Referral Letter / Discharge Summary

> The patient provides a **credible** / *reliable* history of gradual onset of symptoms over the past three months.

Scientific Literature

> A **credible argument** for the existence of quadruplex DNA in vivo is the prevalence of […]. Fry, M. (2007).
>
> Results of this meta-analysis identified more **credible evidence** validating that aromatherapy could significantly decrease labour pain both in early active and late active phases. Liao, C.C. et al. (2021).
>
> Occupational health nurses need to understand tests for COVID-19 infection and antibodies, how to interpret results, and where to find **credible information** and resources. Cadet, M.J. (2020).
>
> A potential problem, however, is that such models, while robust and predictive, may still lack **credibility** from the perspective of the end-user. Spinu, N. et al. (2022).

MEDICAL EDITION

culminate (vi) [B2]

Word family: n: culmination

to reach the highest point or final stage, ending with a specific result or outcome

+ n as subject | process | + prep | in, with

Dialogue

Patient   My years of unhealthy eating habits seem to have finally **culminated in** / *led to* this recent heart attack.

Doctor   Unfortunately I would have to agree. So, let's work on a plan to improve your cardiovascular health.

Q&A

Questioner   How do you envision your research findings influencing clinical practice in the long-term?

Presenter   I believe our findings will ultimately **culminate in** / *led to* more personalised treatment protocols for patients, which will significantly improve outcomes over the next decade.

Informal

Colleague 1   Did you hear about the major breakthrough in our department's cancer research?

Colleague 2   Yes, I did — it's amazing how years of dedicated work can suddenly **culminate** / *result* in such a game-changing discovery!

Referral Letter / Discharge Summary

The patient's worsening symptoms over the past month **culminated in** / *led to* an acute episode of respiratory distress, necessitating emergency department admission. As a **culmination** / *result* **of** our diagnostic efforts, we identified a previously undetected pulmonary embolism as the underlying cause of her deteriorating condition.

Scientific Literature

Translation is controlled mainly during its initiation, a **process** which **culminates in** a ribosome positioned with an initiator tRNA over the start codon and [...]. Querido, J.B. et al. (2024).

Here, we present the basic principles behind these epigenetic pathways and highlight the evidence suggesting that their misregulation can **culminate in** cancer. Dawson, M.A., Kouzarides, T. (2012).

With accelerating greenhouse gas emissions, species losses from warming and oxygen depletion alone become comparable to current direct human impacts within a century and **culminate in** a mass extinction rivaling those in Earth's past. Penn, J.L., Deutsch, C. (2022).

cumulative (adj)

Word family: adv: cumulatively; syn: accumulative

growing in impact or significance with each addition; incorporating all previous additions over time

---

+ n | dose, exposure | effect | impact

Dialogue

Patient   My headaches seem to be getting worse over time, especially with stress.

Doctor   It sounds like you're experiencing **cumulative** / *increasing* strain on your nervous system.

Q&A

Questioner   How did your research account for potential long-term side effects of the treatment?

Presenter   Our longitudinal studies showed that the benefits of the treatment **cumulatively** / *progressively* outweighed the risks over a five-year period.

Informal

Colleague 1   Have you noticed how the **cumulative** / *growing* effect of these late-night grant-writing sessions is really taking a toll on everyone's mood?

Colleague 2   Yeah, I was just thinking we should propose a department-wide week off after the next funding deadline.

Referral Letter / Discharge Summary

> The patient's symptoms have **cumulatively** / *steadily* worsened over the past six months, despite conservative management, necessitating referral to a specialist for further evaluation and potential surgical intervention.

Scientific Literature

> 'The **cumulative effect** of insufficient sleep on adolescent obesity: evidence from a Spanish cohort'. Mitra, S. (2023).
>
> OBJECTIVES: To evaluate the current evidence that **cumulative exposure** to inorganic lead is associated with decreased performance in neurobehavioural tests in adults. Balbus-Kornfeld, J.M. et al. (1995).
>
> Assessing and managing the **cumulative impacts** of human activities on the environment remains a major challenge to sustainable development. Willsteed, E. et al. (2017).
>
> **Cumulative** COVID-19 statistics predicted managers' anxiety and depression symptoms positively, while **non-cumulative** daily COVID-19 statistics predicted anxiety and depression symptoms negatively. Li, L. et al. (2022).

MEDICAL EDITION

debilitate (vt) `C1`

Word family: adj: debilitating; n: debility, debilitation; syn: drain

to weaken the body, mind or strength of a person, group or system

---

(vt, adj) + n | effect | condition | disease, illness | system |
(adj) + prep | to

Dialogue

Patient I haven't slept more than two hours a night for the past three months, and I seem to be constantly ill.

Doctor Your chronic insomnia has probably significantly **debilitated** / *weakened* your **immune system**.

Q&A

Questioner Can you explain how your research addresses the long-term consequences of chronic migraines?

Presenter Our five-year study reveals that untreated migraines have a **debilitating** / *harmful* **effect** on both cognitive function and quality of life.

Informal

Colleague 1 I've been training for a marathon, but these new overnight shifts are really messing with my schedule.

Colleague 2 Yes, constant disruption of your circadian rhythm is **debilitating** / *damaging* **to** both your athletic performance and recovery time.

Referral Letter / Discharge Summary

> The patient's progressive rheumatoid arthritis has severely **debilitated** / *weakened* her hand function recently. This ongoing **debility** / *weakness* significantly impacts her ability to perform essential daily activities, including personal hygiene.

Scientific Literature

> Noise not only affects the auditory system but can also **debilitate** other non-auditory **systems** as evidenced in animal and human models. Arjunan, A., Rajan, R. (2020).
>
> Although the incidence of this lesion has been declining, it still **debilitates** many geriatric patients, especially with neurological or malignant diseases. Kanazawa, K. (1990).
>
> When practice makes imperfect: **debilitating effects** of overlearning (article title). Larger, E.J., Imber, L.G. (1979).
>
> Inherited degenerative diseases of the brain are chronically progressive and often lead to severe **debilitation**. March, P.A. (1996).

ENGLISH EXPRESSIONS IN CONTEXT

deduce (vt)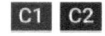

Word family: n: deduction; syn: infer

to conclude or infer (from) something based on available information, evidence or known facts

v + | **be able to** | adv | **logically** | **easily** | + prep | **from**

Dialogue

Patient   I've been feeling really tired and lightheaded recently. Any idea what's causing it?

Doctor   From what you're describing, I'd **deduce** / *think* **that** it could be related to your medication.

Q&A

Questioner   I'm curious about the potential limitations of your study design and how this might impact the generalisability of your conclusions.

Presenter   While there are some limitations, the validity of our data **can** be **deduced** / *seen* **from** the consistency of our results across multiple patient populations.

Informal

Colleague 1   How is the process of buying a new car going? I know you were a bit stuck last time we spoke.

Colleague 2   Based on what I've heard from friends, I have **deduced** / *realised* **that** the best approach is to prioritise my non-negotiables and set my budget.

Referral Letter / Discharge Summary

Upon reviewing the patient's extensive ophthalmological history and gradual visual decline over the past three years, we **can deduce** / *it is clear* **that** the bilateral cataracts are the primary cause of their current symptoms.

Scientific Literature

By understanding the principles of human steroid biosynthesis, the pathogenesis of each disorder may be **logically deduced** [...]. Auchus, R.J., Chang, A.Y. (2010).

The age at which infants can demonstrate the **ability to deduce** abstract rules can be reduced by more than half, from 21 months to 9 months. Diamond, A. (2006).

The ideal clinician knows themselves and their environment, truly observes, imagines the possibilities, **deduces from** what they observe, and continually learns. Gardiner, F.W. (2016).

Application in context

deduce vs induce vs deduct: **deduce** *means to draw a conclusion based on evidence, while* **induce** *refers to causing something to happen or influence a situation. In contrast,* **deduct** *means to subtract or remove a portion of a whole.*

deem (vt)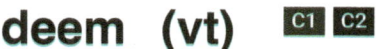

Word family: syn: consider

to consider, judge or hold a specific opinion about somebody/something

+ adj | necessary | proper | crucial | appropriate

Dialogue

Patient My anxiety levels have escalated so much lately that they are now affecting my daily life.

Doctor Based on your symptoms, I would **deem** / *consider* it **necessary** to schedule you for an MRI to rule out any serious underlying conditions.

Q&A

Questioner How do you reconcile the potential side effects of the proposed treatment with its benefits?

Presenter Given the severity of symptoms, I **deem** / *believe* (or *consider*) it **crucial** to prioritise long-term quality of life improvements over short-term discomfort from manageable side effects.

Informal

Colleague 1 Why hasn't the proposal been approved?

Colleague 2 It wasn't **deemed** / *considered* **appropriate** given the current priorities and budget constraints.

Referral Letter / Discharge Summary

It was **deemed necessary** / *essential* to address the patient's cholesterol disparity, as the lipid panel revealed levels that could potentially impact her cardiovascular health.

Scientific Literature

Moral distress occurs when individuals feel powerless to do what they think is right, including when clinicians are prevented from providing health care they **deem necessary**. Rivlin, K. et al. (2024).

Imatinib, the first and arguably the best targeted therapy, became the springboard for developing drugs aimed at molecular targets **deemed crucial** to tumours. Prasad, V. et al. (2016).

Nine viruses had a 'strong' causality score and were **deemed** causal. Edridge, A.W.D., van der Hoek, L. (2020).

ENGLISH EXPRESSIONS IN CONTEXT

deficient (adj) C1

Word family: n: deficiency

lacking sufficient amounts of something, especially something necessary; not meeting the required standard or quality

---

v + | be, become | prove | + prep | in | (n) + adj | iron, dietary

Dialogue

Patient I've been feeling really tired lately and my hair seems to be thinning.

Doctor Based on your symptoms, it's possible **your iron has become deficient** / *you're low on iron*.

Q&A

Questioner How does your research account for genetic factors?

Presenter While genetics play a role, our findings strongly suggest **dietary deficiency** / *poor nutrition* as the primary cause.

Informal

Colleague 1 How's your iron supplementation progressing?

Colleague 2 I've finally overcome my **iron deficiency** / *low iron* after three months of supplements.

Referral Letter / Discharge Summary

Initial assessments proved **deficient** / *fell short* in identifying the underlying cause of the patient's chronic abdominal pain, necessitating further specialised gastrointestinal evaluation.

Scientific Literature

Further insights into their function have come from analyses of mice **deficient in** either cytokine. Ushach, I., Zlotnik, A. (2016).

The elderly may be the most at risk group of suffering dysphagia as well as most likely to be **deficient in** micronutrients. Rodd, B.G. et al. (2022).

[…] there is a major **deficiency** in controlled clinical trials, the conduct of which should be a focus for the near future. Jordan, S.C., Pescovitz, M.D. (2006).

Application in context

Deficient *appears in common medical labels such as 'Attention Deficit Hyperactivity Disorder' (ADHD), and 'Acquired Immunodeficiency Syndrome' (AIDS).*

defy (vt)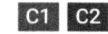

Word family: n: defiance (prep + | in defiance (of)); adj + | blatant, direct, open)

deliberately disobey authority or rules; exceed rational comprehension; resist or withstand remarkably well

+ n as object | common sense, conventional wisdom, the status quo | authority, belief, convention | expectation | imagination | logic, prediction, reason

Dialogue

Patient   I've been feeling better even though I realised I've been taking the wrong pills.

Doctor   That's surprising. It seems to **defy logic** / *not make logical sense*, but it's possible you were getting a placebo effect.

Q&A

Questioner   Your research findings are intriguing, but don't they contradict the current scientific consensus?

Presenter   While our results may **defy the status quo** / *go against accepted beliefs*, our rigorous experiments support our conclusions and warrant further research.

Informal

Colleague 1   Did you attend the keynote speech this morning? The presenter's ideas about the future of medical research seem to **defy imagination** / *seem too incredible to imagine*.

Colleague 2   Absolutely! It was fascinating to hear such a bold and innovative perspective on where our field is headed.

Referral Letter / Discharge Summary

The patient continues to **defy** / *rebel against* medical advice regarding smoking cessation despite multiple counselling sessions. This **defiance** / *refusal* appears rooted in low motivation for change.

Scientific Literature

Some stochastic effects may seem to **defy common sense** but nevertheless they may be very real from the theoretical and practical perspectives. Klebanov, L.B., Yakovlev, A.Y. (2008).

This result **defies conventional wisdom** and suggests that [...]. Fridlind, A.M. et al. (2004).

ENGLISH EXPRESSIONS IN CONTEXT

deplete (vt, vi) `C1`

Word family: n: depletion; syn: consume, exhaust

to significantly use up or reduce a resource, leaving an insufficient amount remaining

+ n as object | **level** | **reserve, resource** | **supply** | **ozone**

Dialogue

Patient I've been feeling incredibly tired lately, with no energy at all.

Doctor Your blood tests indicate your iron levels are severely **depleted** / *low*, which explains your fatigue.

Q&A

Questioner Could you please explain the energy shortfall you observed in the clinical trials?

Presenter Our findings suggest that the new treatment protocol rapidly **depletes** / *uses up* the body's glucose **reserves**, necessitating immediate dietary intervention.

Informal

Colleague 1 I heard you worked a double shift in the ER yesterday – how did it go?

Colleague 2 It was intense. By the end of the day, I was completely **depleted** / *exhausted* from running around nonstop.

Referral Letter / Discharge Summary

> Physical examination revealed severe hyponatremia secondary to **depleted** / *low* sodium **levels** following prolonged vomiting and diarrhea.

Scientific Literature

> Decomposer fungi continually **deplete** the organic **resources** they inhabit, so successful colonization of new resources is a crucial part of their ecology. Boddy, L., Hiscox, J. (2016).
>
> Continued use of petroleum sourced fuels is now widely recognized as unsustainable because of **depleting supplies** and […]. Chisti, Y. (2007).
>
> Stratospheric **ozone depletion** due to chlorofluorocarbons and increased ultraviolet radiation penetration has long been predicted. Coldiron, B.M. (1996).

MEDICAL EDITION

deviate (vi) `C1`

Word family: n: deviation, deviant; adj: deviant

to differ from something; to act or proceed differently than what is usual or expected

+ prep | from | by

Dialogue

Patient I'm really worried that my back pain has got much worse over the past few months.

Doctor Looking at your MRI results, I can see that your spine has begun to **deviate** / *drift* **from** its normal curvature, which explains your symptoms.

Q&A

Questioner Your control group showed significant **deviation** / *difference* **from** expected outcomes. How can you be confident in your conclusions?

Presenter The statistical analysis I presented accounts for this variability through our adjusted p-values and confidence intervals.

Informal

Colleague 1 That new AI chatbot gave some really weird answers when I tested it yesterday.

Colleague 2 Well, it could be a statistical **deviant** in the current generation of language models, which actually makes it fascinating to study.

Referral Letter / Discharge Summary

> Though the patient's blood pressure readings initially appeared to **deviate** / *differ* **from** the typical hypertensive pattern, this **deviation** was later attributed to medication timing inconsistencies during his hospital stay.

Scientific Literature

> To this end, they search for mechanisms that cause human behaviour to **deviate from** what seems to be the rational optimum. Hintze, A., Hertwig, R. (2016).
>
> The **deviated** nose represents a complex cosmetic and functional problem. Septal surgery plays a central role in the successful management of the externally **deviated** nose. Foda, H.M.T. (2005).
>
> Three types of **deviant** sounds were designed to vary in duration. Shiga, T. et al. (2011).
>
> **Deviation from** the matching law reflects an optimal strategy involving learning over multiple timescales (article title). Iigaya, K. et al. (2019).

ENGLISH EXPRESSIONS IN CONTEXT

diminish (vt, vi) C1

Word family: syn: decrease

(vt) to become or make something smaller, weaker or less intense; (vi) to lessen the significance or worth of someone or something

+ n as subject | chance, likelihood | number | + n as object | amount | credibility | effect | impact | importance, influence | level | likelihood | prospect | response | risk | value

Dialogue

Patient Will I ever be able to play the violin again after my hand surgery?

Doctor With proper physical therapy and following our rehabilitation plan, we can significantly **diminish** / *lower* the **risk** of any permanent limitations.

Q&A

Questioner Your data indicate that the **number** of positive cases **diminishes** / *reduces* by approximately 20% with each intervention cycle. Have you considered extending the trial period by another six months?

Presenter Unfortunately, our current funding and IRB* approval only allow us to track outcomes through the end of this year.

Informal

Colleague 1 Do you think we should invite the new member to our brainstorming session?

Colleague 2 I'm worried it might **diminish** / *lessen* our **influence** over the project's creative direction.

Referral Letter / Discharge Summary

The patient's frequent requests for early prescription refills and inconsistent accounts of medication usage may **diminish** / *hurt* his **credibility** regarding pain-management compliance, warranting careful monitoring and a potential substance-abuse evaluation.

Scientific Literature

Pulmonary rehabilitation also **diminishes** the **amount** of hospitalisations and the duration of stay in hospitals. Karrer, W. (2005).

As pelvic surgeons become more confident in their efforts to safeguard the urinary tract, the **chance** of an unrecognized injury causing morbidity will **diminish**. Brubaker, L.T., Wilbanks, G.D. (1991).

Different methodologies are developed to prevent or to **diminish** the **level** of injuries. Oliva, J. (2019).

Higher policy uncertainty and concerns regarding health services will **diminish** the positive **impact** of the lockdown on household health status. Sun, R., Zhao, Y. (2023).

MEDICAL EDITION

discern (vt) `C1`

Word family: adj: discernible, discerning; syn: detect, make out

to perceive or comprehend something not immediately obvious; to detect or notice something, often with effort

---

+ n as object | **meaning** | **pattern** | **truth** | + sub conj | **if, whether** | **which**

Dialogue

Patient I sometimes hear whispering voices and can't tell if they are real or just in my head.

Doctor We need to **discern** / *determine* **whether** these are hallucinations or related to the stress you're currently experiencing.

Q&A

Questioner How did you account for potential environmental factors influencing gene expression in these patients?

Presenter We employed advanced statistical models to **discern** / *separate* genetic influences from environmental factors.

Informal

Colleague 1 I'm hearing mixed reviews of the new sushi place down the street – any advice?

Colleague 2 You can usually **discern** / *tell* a good sushi spot by how they prepare their rice – it's all about the perfect balance of vinegar and sugar.

Referral Letter / Discharge Summary

> After extensive diagnostic testing and clinical observation, we were able to **discern** / *identify* a **pattern** of intermittent tachycardia triggered by specific physical exertions, which may indicate an underlying cardiovascular condition.

Scientific Literature

> Such a synthesis may also help us **discern meaning** inherent in this complex neurobehavioral syndrome. Fricchione, G., Beach, S. (2019).
>
> Semantic MEDLINE provides a roadmap through content and helps users **discern patterns** in large numbers of retrieved citations. Rindflesh, T.C. et al. (2017).
>
> Contrary to a common narrative whereby politics drives susceptibility to fake news, people are 'better' at **discerning truth** from falsehood (despite greater overall belief) when evaluating politically concordant news. Pennycook, G., Rand, D.G. (2021).
>
> No factors were able to **discern which** patients could be evaluated by corrected serum calcium levels. Byrnes, M.C. et al. (2005).

ENGLISH EXPRESSIONS IN CONTEXT

disparity (n) `C1`

Word family: adj: disparate

a noticeable difference, particularly one linked to inequality or unfair treatment

adj + | economic, socio-economic | gender, sex | racial, ethnic |
v + | address, reduce | eliminate | increase

Dialogue

Patient I'm here for my annual check-up.

Doctor Excellent. Based on your test results, we'll discuss any potential health **disparities** / *concerns* that might affect your overall well-being.

Q&A

Questioner Your study shows **disparate** / *different* **outcomes** between urban and rural populations, but have you considered socioeconomic factors?

Presenter Although I didn't have time to elaborate during the presentation, we did account for socioeconomic **disparities** / *differences* in our analysis.

Informal

Colleague 1 Hey, did you catch that documentary on sustainable architecture last night?

Colleague 2 No, I missed it, but I've been noticing a growing **disparity** / *gap* between eco-friendly building practices and what's actually being implemented in our city.

Referral Letter / Discharge Summary

It was deemed necessary to **address** the patient's cholesterol **disparity** / *imbalance* as the lipid panel revealed levels that could potentially impact her cardiovascular health.

Scientific Literature

'**Socio-economic disparity** in visual impairment from cataract'. Fang, Z. et al. (2021).

Gender disparity in plastic surgery in Canada is an important issue. Retrouvey, H., Gdalevitch, P. (2018).

However, two questions await further investigation: whether **disparity** in depression correlated with socioeconomic status will become larger when depression becomes severer, and whether digital technology will **reduce** the **disparity** in depression correlated with socioeconomic status. Mu, A. et al. (2021).

MEDICAL EDITION

disrupt (vt) C1

Word family: n: disruption (v + | cause, create, lead to);
adj: disruptive (+ n | event | behaviour)

to interfere with or disturb the normal flow or operation of something

+ n as object | sleep | balance, process | system

Dialogue

Patient   I've been feeling quite unwell lately, with persistent fatigue, digestive issues and mood swings.

Doctor   It seems that certain lifestyle factors may be **disrupting** / *upsetting* the delicate **balance** of your physical and mental well-being.

Q&A

Questioner   Do you think this novel therapeutic approach will **disrupt** / *change* the current standard of care for patients?

Presenter   Obviously, further research is needed to fully assess the impact on existing treatment protocols.

Informal

Colleague 1   Did you catch the keynote speech on how artificial intelligence is poised to **disrupt** / *revolutionise* the way we diagnose and treat rare genetic disorders?

Colleague 2   It was absolutely mind-blowing to see how machine learning algorithms can help our expertise.

Referral Letter / Discharge Summary

Chronic pain has continued to **disrupt** / *disturb* the patient's sleep, with frequent nighttime awakenings reported. This ongoing **sleep disruption** / *lack of sleep* (or *insomnia*) has led to daytime fatigue, poor concentration and increased irritability.

Scientific Literature

There is growing evidence that environmental chemicals can **disrupt** endocrine **systems**. Boas, M. et al. (2006).

The Covid-19 pandemic has been the highest **disruptive event** in the world recent history. Fassin, Y. (2021).

Thus, mutations in MED12 can **cause disruption** of CDK8 kinase activity through two separate mechanisms. Gonzalez, C.G. et al. (2022).

ENGLISH EXPRESSIONS IN CONTEXT

distort (vt) C1

Word family: n: distortion

to modify something's form, sound or look, making it unclear or unnatural; to misrepresent information, altering its truth or accuracy

+ n as object | history | meaning | memory, perception | reality, truth

Dialogue

Patient   I've been feeling so anxious lately, I can't think clearly.

Doctor   Anxiety can sometimes **distort** / *change* your **perception** of situations, making things feel worse than they actually are. Let's work on some strategies to help manage it.

Q&A

Questioner   Your results seem to **distort** / *alter* the **meaning** of the original hypothesis, given that you excluded patients over 65.

Presenter   Actually, we maintained strict adherence to the original hypothesis by focusing on the working-age population, as specified in our pre-registered protocol.

Informal

Colleague 1   The social media post makes it look like we changed our entire approach.

Colleague 2   They totally **distorted** / *misrepresented* our message to make it clickbait.

Referral Letter / Discharge Summary

> The patient's anxiety tends to **distort** / *alter* her **perception** of physical symptoms, though this cognitive **distortion** / *misinterpretation* has improved with the combination of sertraline and CBT*.

Scientific Literature

> There are growing concerns about the potential for deepfake technology to spread misinformation and **distort memories** [...]. Murphy, G. et al. (2023).

> Whatever its intuitive appeal, the psychological concept of dehumanization might do more to **distort** than illuminate the **history** of collective violence. Lang, J. (2020).

> The results indicate that when the body's truth is filtered through intersectional lenses, this **truth** can become **distorted** or lost. León-Menjivar, C.D. (2022).

diverge (vi) `C2`

Word family: n: divergence; adj: divergent

to move or branch off in different directions; to differ in opinions or views; to deviate from what is anticipated or intended

+ prep | from

Dialogue

Patient   I keep having the same symptoms over and over again.

Doctor   Your case appears to **diverge** / *seems different* **from** the typical pattern we usually observe in these situations.

Q&A

Questioner   Have you considered how your findings might be explained by age-related changes in metabolism?

Presenter   Yes, and that's precisely why we see such **divergent** / *different* outcomes between our younger and older patient cohorts.

Informal

Colleague 1   Looking back at your career, which do you think was more influential, luck or planning?

Colleague 2   I'd say it was the small daily choices we made that led us to our **divergent** / *different* paths.

Referral Letter / Discharge Summary

The patient's clinical course continued to **diverge** / *differ* **from** our initial expectations, as her symptoms worsened despite appropriate antibiotic therapy.

Scientific Literature

Drawing on research from clinical, physiological, and other subfields of psychology, they show that emotional reactions to risky situations often **diverge from** cognitive assessments of those risks. When such **divergence** occurs, emotional reactions often drive behaviour. Loewenstein, G.F. et al. (2001).

As populations **diverge**, genetic differences accumulate across the genome. Wolf, J.B.W., Ellegren, H. (2017).

This could possibly represent differentially methylated sites that have caused **divergent** genetic mutations between species, or **divergent** selection leading to both genetic and epigenetic variation at these sites. Venney, C.J. et al. (2024).

ENGLISH EXPRESSIONS IN CONTEXT

efficacy (n)

Word family: adj: efficacious; adv: efficaciously; syn: effectiveness

the capability of something to achieve its intended outcome; the performance of a treatment or drug in controlled scientific trials

+ prep | against | at, in, of | to

Dialogue

Patient These antibiotics you prescribed aren't working well enough for my sinus infection.

Doctor I'm confident that this medication will clear your infection soon based on recent studies showing excellent **efficacy** / *success* **against** this particular bacterial strain.

Q&A

Questioner Why did you choose this specific drug combination for your clinical trial?

Presenter Our preliminary lab studies demonstrated remarkable **efficacy** / *power* **to** eliminate resistant bacteria, which led us to test this combination in patients.

Informal

Colleague 1 Looks like it's going to rain all weekend – there go my hiking plans!

Colleague 2 Actually, I've found hiking in light rain can be surprisingly **efficacious** / *helpful* in clearing my mind after a long week in the clinic.

Referral Letter / Discharge Summary

The patient's renal function has improved steadily, demonstrating the high **efficacy** / *effectiveness* **of** the adjusted diuretic regimen.

Scientific Literature

Conventional paired meta-analyses have shown inconsistent results regarding the safety and **efficacy of** different interventions. Wei, F.L. et al. (2021).

Numerous studies on pharmacologic treatments and non-pharmacologic therapies for constipation have attempted to overcome limitations such as temporary and insufficient **efficacy**. Ryu, H.S., Choi, S.C. (2015).

T cells can **efficaciously** control HIV replication, and it has been hypothesized that inducing those responses before exposure occurs may prevent HIV infection. Streeck, H. (2016).

Application in context

efficacy vs. efficiency: **efficacy** *refers to how well a treatment achieves its intended medical outcome, while* **efficiency** *refers to how well time, money, and resources are utilised in the delivery. See page 110.*

MEDICAL EDITION

efficient (adj)

Word family n: efficiency

performing tasks thoroughly and properly without wasting time, resources or energy

+ n | administration, management | means, method, way | organisation

Dialogue

Patient — I've been trying to manage my symptoms, but it feels like I'm not making progress.

Doctor — Right, let's find a more **efficient** / *helpful* **way** to help you cope, so you don't feel like you are wasting time and energy and getting nowhere.

Q&A

Questioner — How did you decide which testing algorithm to use for screening the high-risk patients?

Presenter — We selected this **method** for its **efficiency** / *how well it works* because it reduced false positives while keeping costs manageable.

Informal

Colleague 1 — Our emergency department's **efficiency** / *speed and quality* has really improved since we implemented the new triage protocol!

Colleague 2 — The patients definitely seem happier now that their wait times are shorter.

Referral Letter / Discharge Summary

While Mr. Johnson's **efficient** / *quick* **response** to the new medication helped us achieve peak treatment **efficiency** / *quality*, we recommend continued monitoring by his primary care physician.

Scientific Literature

A comprehensive understanding of the different molecular mechanisms [...] may be an **efficient means** to improve its clinical efficacy in the future. Liu, L. et al. (2023).

This is the first of a series of six articles which [...] will demonstrate that **efficient** practice **management** is not only desirable, but also achievable. Wilkinson, M.D. (1989).

Emergency department (ED) operations leaders are under increasing pressure to make care delivery more **efficient**. Publicly reported ED **efficiency** metrics are traditionally patient centred [...]. Heaton, H.A. et al. (2020).

Application in context

efficient vs. effective: **efficient** *relates to the optimal use of time, money, and resources in treatment delivery, while* **effective** *refers to the ability to achieve the intended medical outcome. See page* **110**.

ENGLISH EXPRESSIONS IN CONTEXT

elicit (vt)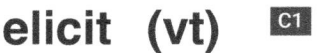

Word family: n: elicitation

to obtain information or a response from someone, often with effort

+ n | comment | information | reaction, reply, response, criticism | emotion, sympathy

Dialogue

Patient   The treatment doesn't seem to be working – nothing's really changed.

Doctor   If that's the case, we'll try an alternative approach to **elicit** / *provoke* a more effective **response** and better address your symptoms.

Q&A

Questioner   Your surprising findings about patient recovery rates in the control group have **elicited** / *caused* **criticism** from several of my colleagues who reported different outcomes.

Presenter   Our methodology carefully controlled for age and comorbidity factors, which may explain the difference from previous studies.

Informal

Colleague 1   I heard you just adopted a retired lab dog and gave him a forever home.

Colleague 2   His gentle nature, coupled with the scars from past experiments, truly **elicited** / *stirred* my **sympathy**.

Referral Letter / Discharge Summary

The **elicitation** / *gathering* of detailed psychiatric symptoms during the initial consultation revealed a complex pattern of anxiety and depression requiring specialised follow-up care.

Scientific Literature

Complications associated with vaping are newly emerging and relatively unstudied; little guidance exists on how clinicians may best **elicit information** related to vaping practices and associated medical problems. Boyer, E.W. et al. (2020).

One prevalent explanation suggests that perceiving emotional expressions induces emotions in the observer and that it is these emotions that **elicit** the facial **reactions**. This study directly tested this hypothesis, investigating whether **emotion elicitation** is what drives the effect. Shaham, G., Aviezer, H. (2022).

Tasting sweet food **elicits** insulin release prior to increasing plasma glucose levels, known as cephalic phase insulin release (CPIR). Tonosaki, K. et al. (2007).

MEDICAL EDITION

eliminate (vt)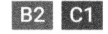

Word family: n: elimination

to remove or get rid of someone or something completely, especially if it is unwanted or unnecessary

+ n | barrier, problem, risk, threat | chance, possibility, uncertainty | effect, influence

Dialogue

Patient   I'm worried about this lump I've found under my armpit.

Doctor   Let's run some tests to **eliminate** / *remove* any **uncertainty** and get a clear diagnosis.

Q&A

Questioner   How did you control for potential confounding variables in your study?

Presenter   We used a randomised controlled design to **eliminate** / *rule out* the **influence** of external factors on our results.

Informal

Colleague 1   This new protocol should **eliminate** / *solve* the **problem** of inconsistent sample storage temperatures.

Colleague 2   Actually, I just finished testing a solar-powered cooling unit that maintains a steady −8°C, even during power outages.

Referral Letter / Discharge Summary

> The thorough diagnostic workup and subsequent treatment have successfully **eliminated** / *ruled out* the **risk** of acute coronary syndrome in this patient.

Scientific Literature

> This article outlines strategies for reducing the stigma and **eliminating** the **barriers** associated with obtaining the mental and emotional well-being support and services that nurses need and deserve. Weston, M.J., Nordberg, A. (2022).
>
> Sperm selection based on viability and normal morphology does not **eliminate** the **chance** for DNA damaged spermatozoa to be inseminated [...]. Nasr-Esfahani, M.H. et al. (2012).
>
> The search for an effective medication that will **eliminate** tinnitus has a long history. Bauer, C.A. (2020).
>
> [...] however, complete **elimination** of sudden cardiac death still remains an elusive gain. Shah, M. (2017).

ENGLISH EXPRESSIONS IN CONTEXT

empirical (adj)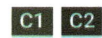

Word family: adv: empirically; n: empiricism, empiric; ant: theoretical

derived from practical observation or experimentation rather than theoretical reasoning or abstract principles

+ n | data | evidence, basis | research | test

Dialogue

Patient Can I expect a positive outcome if I follow your recommendations?

Doctor My approach is based on **empirical evidence** / *experimental data* so there's a high chance it'll work.

Q&A

Questioner How do you propose to validate your findings in real-world scenarios?

Presenter We plan to conduct extensive clinical trials to gather **evidence empirically** / *concrete evidence* from real-world observations and data to support our conclusions.

Informal

Colleague 1 Have you considered any theoretical frameworks for interpreting your research findings?

Colleague 2 Yes, we've developed some theoretical models, but now we're focusing on gathering **empirical data** / *real-world evidence* and observations to test their validity.

Referral Letter / Discharge Summary

The recommended treatment protocol has a strong **empirical basis** / *evidence base* from multiple controlled trials involving over 500 patients with similar presenting symptoms.

Scientific Literature

We use **empirical data** from 24,678 people living in 176 villages in rural Honduras. Ghasemian, A., Christakis, N.A. (2023).

In an analysis of over 350 studies published between 2018 and 2020, we detect **empirical evidence** of exaggeration bias and selective reporting [...]. Kimmel, K. et al. (2023).

Herein, we review the current evidence on nicotine reduction and discuss some of the challenges in establishing the **empirical basis** for regulatory decisions. Donny, E.C. et al. (2014).

Application in context

empirical vs. theoretical: while **empirical knowledge** *comes from direct observation and experience*, **theoretical knowledge** *comes from reasoning and principles. In medical research papers, one often encounters phrases like 'empirical evidence' contrasted with 'theoretical framework'.*

MEDICAL EDITION

endure (vt, vi)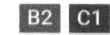

Word family: adj: enduring, endurable; n: endurance

to withstand pain or hardship without giving up; (vi) to persist or last for an extended period

---

+ n as object | **pain, stress, suffering** | **treatment** | **conditions** | **agony, hardship, misery**

Dialogue

Patient   My back has been hurting terribly for six weeks now, especially in the mornings.

Doctor   I'm sorry you've had to **endure** / *deal with* this **pain** for all this time. I believe we should start with an MRI to determine the exact cause.

Q&A

Questioner   How did your patient population respond to the experimental protocol over the trial period?

Presenter   While most patients were able to **endure** / *handle* the **treatment** through completion, we did see a 15% dropout rate.

Informal

Colleague 1   I heard you finally completed the trek to Machu Picchu last month – how was the experience?

Colleague 2   The views were absolutely worth every **hardship** we had to **endure** / *face* during the four-day hike.

Referral Letter / Discharge Summary

> The elderly patient had to **endure** / *bear* poor living **conditions** following her spouse's death, including significant nutritional deficits and social isolation. She now shows **enduring** / *persistent* signs of depression.

Scientific Literature

> The opportunistic pathogen Enterococcus faecium colonizes humans and a wide range of animals, **endures** numerous **stresses**, resists antibiotic treatment and [...]. Wei, Y. et al. (2024).

> When the aims would be equally well served by **enduring suffering** and relieving it, the latter appears to be the preferable option, given that the distress a patient experiences has no positive intrinsic value. Varelius, J. (2019).

> The substantial and **enduring** cognitive **symptom** are not alleviated by medication and causes difficulties in everyday life activities. Lundin, L., Flyckt, L. (2015).

enhance (vt)

Word family: n: enhancement; adj: enhanced

to make something better or more valuable in quality, importance or effectiveness

+ n | effect, effectiveness, efficacy, efficiency | function | health, well-being | knowledge, learning, understanding | ability | quality

Dialogue

Patient The medication you prescribed isn't helping my symptoms at all.

Doctor Let me switch you to a different drug that should **enhance** / *boost* the **effect** of your treatment.

Q&A

Questioner Have you considered how your proposed drug might interact with the liver's metabolic pathways?

Presenter Our preliminary data shows that rather than interfering with liver metabolism, this compound actually **enhances** / *improves* the **function** of key detoxification enzymes.

Informal

Colleague 1 I just signed up for that online Spanish course you mentioned last week!

Colleague 2 That's great – learning a new language really **enhances** / *expands* your **ability** to make new neural connections in the brain.

Referral Letter / Discharge Summary

Mr. Johnson's adherence to the prescribed physiotherapy regimen has significantly **enhanced** / *improved* his respiratory **function**.

Scientific Literature

Drug delivery systems (DDS) have improved therapeutic agent administration by **enhancing efficacy** and patient compliance while minimizing side effects. Abbasi, M. et al. (2024).

We developed a weekly transdermal delivery system (TDS) for the sustained delivery of RLX (Raloxifene) to **enhance** the therapeutic **effectiveness**, increase adherence, and reduce side effects. Vora, D. et al (2022).

Courses that teach evidence-based interventions to **enhance well-being** are a public health tool that could be used to improve mental health in the population. Yaden, D.B. et al. (2021).

'Can citizen science **enhance** public **understanding** of science?' Bonney, R. et al. (2016).

MEDICAL EDITION

ensue (vi)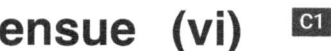

Word family: adj: ensuing

to occur following or as a consequence of a previous event

+ n as subject | argument, discussion | conflict, fight, fighting, struggle | silence | chaos | trouble

Dialogue

Patient   I started the new medication yesterday, but I felt dizzy soon after.

Doctor   Side effects can sometimes **ensue** / *follow* when starting this treatment. Let's monitor it closely and adjust if needed.

Q&A

Questioner   Your findings seem to contradict the famous report published last year by the French team – are you not worried about the backlash that may **ensue** / *arise*?

Presenter   I acknowledge the considerable discrepancy and hope that it'll give rise to a productive argument.

Informal

Colleague 1   Did you hear about the debate in yesterday's meeting?

Colleague 2   I did. A heated discussion **ensued** / *followed* after they brought up the budget cuts.

Referral Letter / Discharge Summary

A significant **struggle ensued** / *occurred* as the patient attempted to maintain his balance during ambulation*, necessitating an immediate referral to physical therapy.

Scientific Literature

As people age, gradual changes **ensue** in vision, hearing, balance, coordination, and memory. Farage, M.A. et al. (2012).

Joint and muscle injury associated with direct damage to the tissues and muscle atrophy may **ensue** following immobility. Buzzard, B.M. (1998).

Ultimately, the **conflicts** that **ensue** from dreaming during crisis generate possibilities of learning through crisis. Neufeld, M. (2021).

ENGLISH EXPRESSIONS IN CONTEXT

equitable (adj)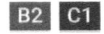

Word family: n: equity; adj: equitably; ant: inequitable; syn: fair, just

just and impartial, treating all individuals equally

+ n | access | distribution | health, health care, health system | life | system

Dialogue

Patient   I can't sleep at night due to constant coughing.

Doctor   An **equitable*** / *sensible* course of action is to start with testing for allergies and acid reflux.

Q&A

Questioner   How do your findings about diabetes treatments account for socioeconomic disparities in patient access?

Presenter   Our research shows that digital monitoring combined with community health workers helps patients across all income levels achieve a more **equitable** / *fairer* **life**.

Informal

Colleague 1   I really miss having time to read novels since starting my research fellowship.

Colleague 2   You might find that listening to audiobooks during your commute is an **equitable** / *reasonable* substitute for traditional reading.

Referral Letter / Discharge Summary

An **equitable** / *balanced* **care** plan has been developed incorporating both hospital and community services.

Scientific Literature

We examine the factors that challenge **equitable access** to these novel therapies across minoritized racial, ethnic, and socioeconomic populations. Holstein, S.A. et al. (2023).

The rapid development of coronavirus disease 2019 (COVID-19) vaccines has not been met with the assurance of an effective and **equitable** global **distribution** mechanism. Binagwaho, A. et al. (2022).

The need for an **equitable system** where all women are either notified or not, and also provided with publicly funded supplemental screening was raised by GPs. Nickel, B. et al. (2021).

eradicate (vt)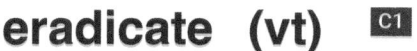

Word family: n: eradication; syn: wipe out

to completely eliminate or destroy something harmful or undesirable

+ n | disease | poverty | disparity, prejudice, a specific disease, such as smallpox

Dialogue

Patient   I've been taking the antibiotics you prescribed for my H. pylori infection, but I'm not sure that they're working.

Doctor   The latest test results show we've successfully **eradicated** / *cleared* the bacteria from your stomach.

Q&A

Questioner   What would you say is the most significant challenge in dealing with antimicrobial-resistant tuberculosis in rural settings?

Presenter   While our new treatment protocol shows promise, we must acknowledge that it's unlikely to completely **eradicate** / *wipe out* drug-resistant TB strains without also addressing poverty and access to healthcare in these regions.

Informal

Colleague 1   Did you try that new pest control service for your garden that I recommended?

Colleague 2   Yes, and they managed to completely **eradicate** / *get rid of* the ant problem that was ruining my patio!

Referral Letter / Discharge Summary

Following completion of the prescribed six-month isoniazid and rifampicin regimen, we have successfully **eradicated** / *cleared* the pulmonary tuberculosis infection, as confirmed by three consecutive negative sputum cultures.

Scientific Literature

Current treatment does not **eradicate** disease, and therefore new treatments are urgently needed. Cargill, T., Barnes, E. (2021).

The cascade of events started with the development of polio vaccines and the realization that polio, much like **smallpox**, could be **eradicated**. Mohammed, A. et al. (2021).

As health professionals, researchers, educators, and leaders, we have a responsibility to take action to **eradicate** racism from the healthcare system. Dhaliwal, R. et al. (2022).

To cure a patient's cancer is to **eradicate** invasive cells from the ecosystem of the body. Noorbakhsh, J. et al. (2020).

ENGLISH EXPRESSIONS IN CONTEXT

erroneous (adj)

Word family: n: error; adv: erroneously

incorrect or mistaken

+ n | **assumption | conclusion | information | perception**

Dialogue

Patient I looked up my symptoms online – I have a migraine.

Doctor The internet features a lot of **erroneous** / *incorrect* **information** about migraines – it's not advisable to self-diagnose this condition.

Q&A

Questioner Couldn't your findings be attributed to potentially confounding variables?

Presenter We believe the relationship isn't **erroneous** / *mistaken* because we did control for the most obvious confounding variables.

Informal

Colleague 1 Have you tried that new AI-powered diagnostic tool everyone's been talking about at the conference?

Colleague 2 I haven't, but I heard it **erroneously** / *incorrectly* flagged a high percentage of benign moles as potentially cancerous in the initial trials.

Referral Letter / Discharge Summary

Mrs. Johnson's initial **erroneous** / *incorrect* **perception** that her symptoms were due to food allergies led to a delay in seeking appropriate medical attention for her gastrointestinal issues, which were later diagnosed as early-stage colorectal cancer.

Scientific Literature

While analyzing data extracted from our EMR for a retrospective study, we identified various types of **erroneous** data entries. Baier, A.W. et al. (2017).

This approach is based in an **erroneous assumption** of equality between men and women. Ruiz-Cantero, M., Verdú-Delgado, M. (2004).

Experience shows that reliance of noninvasive methods led to the **erroneous conclusion** that some subjects were not infected. Graham, D.Y. (2024).

Many health professionals and patients **erroneously** believe that professional ethics and laws protect the privacy of sensitive records in obstetrics-gynecology. Rothstein, M.A. (2023).

MEDICAL EDITION

exacerbate (vt) C1

Word family: n: exacerbation; syn: aggravate

to worsen a condition or problem, making it more severe

+ n | condition, problem, situation | symptom | anxiety

Dialogue

Patient I've noticed that running seems to **exacerbate** / *worsen* my health **problems**.

Doctor Let's explore some alternative exercises that might be gentler on your body.

Q&A

Questioner How do lifestyle factors impact the course of this illness?

Presenter Our data indicates that poor sleep patterns and high-stress environments can **exacerbate** / *worsen* the **situation**, leading to more frequent symptom flare-ups.

Informal

Colleague 1 Did you hear about the new deadline for the quarterly report?

Colleague 2 Yeah, and the shortened time frame is really going to **exacerbate** / *increase* my **anxiety** about getting everything done on time.

Referral Letter / Discharge Summary

The patient reports that prolonged sitting tends to **exacerbate** / *worsen* her lower-back **condition**, particularly during long working hours. Given the frequency of **exacerbation** / *worsening symptoms* in the workplace setting, occupational therapy assessment is strongly recommended.

Scientific Literature

Heat and sweating are thought to especially **exacerbate** itch. Murota, H., Katayama, I. (2017).

The role of infection in asthma is varied in that it may **exacerbate** established asthma or contribute to the initial development of the clinical onset of asthma. Darveaux, J.I., Lemanske Jr. R.F. (2014).

Although pulmonary embolism (PE) can **exacerbate** respiratory **symptoms** such as dyspnea and chest pain [...]. Rizkallah, J. et al. (2009).

The effects of chocolate on acne **exacerbations** have recently been reevaluated. Vongraviopap, S., Asawanonda, P. (2016).

Application in context

exacerbate vs. aggrvate: **exacerbate** *refers to making a medical condition or symptoms worse, while* **aggravate** *traditionally means to irritate or annoy. See page* **111**.

ENGLISH EXPRESSIONS IN CONTEXT

explicit (adj)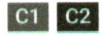

Word family: adv: explicitly; ant: implicit

clearly expressed and unambiguous, leaving no room for misinterpretation; speaking directly, precisely and openly

+ prep | about, as to | + n | denial | memory | statement | policy

Dialogue

Patient I'm not sure I fully understand the side effects of the medication.

Doctor Let me be more **explicit** / *clear* **about** common side effects. These include nausea, dizziness and fatigue, but they should subside after a few days.

Q&A

Questioner How does your research address the potential long-term side effects of this new treatment?

Presenter Our study includes an **explicit** / *detailed* follow-up **protocol** designed to monitor patients for a five-year period post-treatment, allowing us to track any emerging long-term effects.

Informal

Colleague 1 Did you see someone took my lunch from the break room fridge?

Colleague 2 That's terrible. Although it seems obvious, I think we now need an **explicit** / *clear* **policy** about labeling our food containers.

Referral Letter / Discharge Summary

The patient's **explicit** / *insistent* **denial** of any alcohol consumption contradicts the liver function test results, suggesting a need for further investigation into potential substance use.

Scientific Literature

In this review, we investigate particularities of the relationship between **explicit** and implicit **memories** in Alzheimer's disease (AD). Machado, S. et al. (2009).

A decline in declarative or **explicit memory** has been extensively characterized in cognitive aging and is a hallmark of cognitive impairments. Zhivago, K.A. et al. (2020).

Unlike traditional narrative reviews, meta-analyses require **explicit statement** of the criteria for the review and hence highlight these difficulties. Jones, D.R. (1992).

Explicitly obtaining consent from a patient prior to starting a sensitive physical exam is essential to improve their experience with intimate examinations such as the genitourinary exam. Keller, J.M. (2019).

MEDICAL EDITION

extract (vt, n)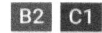

Word family: n: extraction; adj: extractable

a concentrated substance obtained through a specific process; a brief section from a larger work, offering a sample of its content

+ n | cell | information | + prep | from

Dialogue

Patient I've been having this terrible toothache for the past week and can barely sleep at night.

Doctor Looking at your X-ray, we'll need to **extract** / *remove* **from** that back tooth the infected nerve tissue that's causing your pain.

Q&A

Questioner Have you considered how your research on COVID-19 antibodies might apply to other respiratory viruses?

Presenter Yes, the patterns we could **extract from** / *identify in* our longitudinal antibody data suggest similar immune responses might occur with influenza and RSV* infections.

Informal

Colleague 1 I heard you picked up beekeeping recently – how's that going?

Colleague 2 It's amazing – I managed to **extract** / *collect* three jars of honey **from** my first harvest last weekend!

Referral Letter / Discharge Summary

Following successful bone marrow **extraction** / *removal* **from** the right iliac crest, the patient remained stable and was discharged with appropriate pain management.

Scientific Literature

A cytobrush was used to **extract cells from** the external parts of the cervix and transferred to 10ml of preservative solution. Pfeifer, I. et al. (2016).

Here, we review common data visualisation and analysis methods used to **extract information from** chemistry data. Segall, M. et al. (2015).

We studied an eco-friendly **extraction** process to obtain an SFN-rich **extract from** broccoli. González, F. et al. (2021).

Application in context

extract vs. collect: **extract** implies removing something embedded within something else using force or special techniques, whilst **collect** involves gathering readily accessible items.

ENGLISH EXPRESSIONS IN CONTEXT

extrapolate (vt, vi)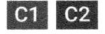

Word family: n: extrapolation

to estimate or form an opinion based on current relevant facts, assuming they apply to a different or future situation

+ n | findings, results | data, values | trend | + prep | from, to

Dialogue

Patient My knee pain has been getting worse over the past few months, and I'm worried about how it might affect me in the future.

Doctor Based on your current progress, we can't directly **extrapolate** / *guess* long-term outcomes, but we'll monitor your condition closely to adjust your treatment as needed.

Q&A

Questioner How confident are you in applying these findings from this sample to the broader patient population?

Presenter Despite the limited sample size, we believe the **trend** observed in our cohort can be reasonably **extrapolated** / *applied* **to** similar patient groups.

Informal

Colleague 1 Did you see the latest sales figures for our new medical textbook?

Colleague 2 Yes, and if we **extrapolate from** / *based on* these numbers, we might double the expected sales.

Referral Letter / Discharge Summary

Given the patient's rapid improvement over the past week, we can **extrapolate** / *predict* that she will likely regain full mobility within the next month, barring any unforeseen complications.

Scientific Literature

It is erroneous to **extrapolate from** events at the level of the neuron or gene to wholescale functions and dysfunctions. Greenfield, S. (1998).

Although the data are thought-provoking, we may not be able to **extrapolate findings** in single dog breeds to the entire species. Smith, A.N. (2014).

It is difficult to **extrapolate data** obtained in experimental animals, as clear species differences exist […]. Chagin, A.S., Savendahl, L. (2007).

Therefore, this paper first uses spline fitting to supplement the missing data and then uses dynamic models to predict the species mortality of the Chinese population, including age **extrapolation** and **trend extrapolation**. Cheng, Z. et al. (2022).

MEDICAL EDITION

feasible (adj) [C1]

Word family: n: feasibility

possible to achieve or successfully carry out

+ v | appear | + adv | barely, entirely, readily | technically | + n | proposition | solution

Dialogue

Patient — I'm usually very active and busy, and am desperate to get rid of this pain in my knee. How often should I do my physical therapy for maximum results?

Doctor — Based on your lifestyle, physical therapy three times a week for six weeks seems like a **feasible** / *achievable* treatment plan to start with. Consistency beats intensity in these cases.

Q&A

Questioner — Could you comment on the **feasibility** / *practicality* of implementing your novel surgical technique in smaller hospitals?

Presenter — While the procedure does require specialised equipment, we've designed a training programme and cost-sharing model that makes it accessible even to smaller facilities.

Informal

Colleague 1 — I can't believe how expensive it's getting to rent a place near the hospital these days.

Colleague 2 — Actually, carpooling with other residents has proven to be a **feasible** / *workable* **solution** for some of our new team members.

Referral Letter / Discharge Summary

Regarding Mr. X's condition, we believe that surgical intervention is **technically feasible** / *possible* given the latest imaging results. However, given his comorbidities, we will conduct further testing to better assess the **feasibility of our options** / *how practical our options are*.

Scientific Literature

In 1969 WHO recommended that, although eradication should remain an ultimate goal, malaria control operations may form a transitional phase in countries where eradication does not **appear feasible**. Sogunro, R. (1993).

Traditional genetic manipulation methods, such as homologous recombination, however, are inefficient, time-consuming, and **barely feasible** when disrupting multiple genes simultaneously. Shi, Y. et al. (2022).

It was demonstrated that a single European database is a **feasible proposition**. Gill, P. et al. (2003).

ENGLISH EXPRESSIONS IN CONTEXT

firsthand (adj, adv)

Word family: adv: firsthand; ant: secondhand

directly experienced or obtained by oneself rather than learned from others or secondary sources

+ n | account | experience | evidence | information, observation | knowledge | report | insight

Dialogue

Patient Doctor, my son has been experiencing these terrible headaches that start at the base of his skull and radiate forward.

Doctor That's very helpful, but I'd like to hear your child's **firsthand** / *personal* **account** of how he's feeling – to make sure we haven't missed anything.

Q&A

Questioner Based on your clinical experience, what are your **firsthand** / *direct* **observations** of patients with multiple conditions?

Presenter I've found that patients with multiple conditions tend to show more variable treatment responses.

Informal

Colleague 1 How was the volunteer medical camp in the countryside?

Colleague 2 I got some great **firsthand** / *direct* **insights** from the lead researcher on treating snake bites.

Referral Letter / Discharge Summary

The patient's partner, who witnessed the seizure **firsthand** / *directly*, reported that it lasted approximately three minutes and was accompanied by tongue-biting and loss of bladder control.

Scientific Literature

Therefore, we focused on the condition of the heart, and sought to provide **firsthand evidence** for whether myocarditis and myocardial injury were caused by COVID-19. Deng, Q. et al. (2020).

Humans rely on communicated information, sometimes even when it contradicts blatantly their **firsthand experience**. Mascaro, O., Kovács, Á.M. (2022).

In this narrative medicine essay, a palliative medicine physician learns **firsthand** how to listen to her mother's end-of-life wishes amid the waves of loss and the noise of the treatment options being offered. Bridges, C. (2023).

Application in context

*While **secondhand** can mean the opposite of 'firsthand,' it more often describes something previously owned by someone else (e.g. second-hand clothes).*

MEDICAL EDITION

heterogeneous (adj)

Word family: n: heterogeneity; adv: heterogeneously

composed of diverse or varied components

+ n | collection, group | disease | population | system

Dialogue

Patient   I've had these strange spots appear on my legs over the past few weeks.

Doctor   The **heterogeneous** / *mixed and varied* nature of these lesions suggests we should do a biopsy to rule out any concerning conditions.

Q&A

Questioner   How did you consider the effect of your patients' different socioeconomic and ethnic backgrounds on your treatment outcomes?

Presenter   Our statistical analysis accounted for this **heterogeneous** / *diverse* **population** through careful stratification of the demographic subgroups.

Informal

Colleague 1   I can't believe how many different streaming services we need these days just to watch our favourite shows!

Colleague 2   Yeah, it's becoming such a **heterogeneous** / *fragmented* landscape of platforms that I finally created a spreadsheet just to track which shows are where.

Referral Letter / Discharge Summary

> The patient's abdominal ultrasound revealed a **heterogeneous** / *mixed texture* liver mass in segment VII measuring 4.2cm in diameter. Given this lesion's **heterogeneity** / *varied appearance* and its concerning features, an urgent MRI with contrast is recommended for further characterisation.

Scientific Literature

> Cervical adenocarcinomas are a **heterogeneous group** of tumours with varying morphologies, aetiologies, molecular drivers, and prognoses*, comprising approximately 25% of all cervical cancers. Hodgson, A., Park, K.J. (2019).
>
> Patients with psoriasis represent a **heterogeneous population** with individual disease expression – different degrees and severity of skin involvement. Dopytalska, K. et al. (2018).
>
> Our understanding of monocytes has advanced from viewing these cells as a homogenous population to a **heterogeneous system** of cells that display diverse responses to different stimuli. Olingy, C.E. et al. (2019).

homogenous (adj)

Word family: n: homogeneity; adv: homogeneously; vt: homogenise

made up of similar or identical elements; consisting of uniform parts or qualities

+ n | group | whole

Dialogue

Patient — I've been having these strange spots appearing all over my body that itch terribly at night.

Doctor — The distribution pattern appears quite **homogeneous** / *evenly spread out*, which, combined with your description of nocturnal itching, strongly suggests scabies*.

Q&A

Questioner — Why did you choose to exclude type B lymphocytes from your experimental design?

Presenter — Since our pilot study showed a **homogeneous** / *uniform* response pattern across all B cell subtypes, we focused our resources on investigating the more variable T cell populations.

Informal

Colleague 1 — Did you try that new Vietnamese restaurant that opened next to the research institute?

Colleague 2 — No, I'm hesitant because the online reviews are so **homogeneous** / *one-sided* – everyone just raves about the pho but nobody mentions any other dishes.

Referral Letter / Discharge Summary

The CT scan revealed a **homogeneous** / *uniform* mass in the left upper lobe measuring 3.2cm x 2.8cm. The lesion's **homogeneity** / *consistency* and well-defined borders suggest a benign aetiology.

Scientific Literature

Classification criteria should only be applied to patients with an established diagnosis and aimed at the identification of a rather **homogeneous group** of patients for the conduction of clinical research. Poddubnyy, D. (2020).

Unlike other methods that treat noise as a **homogeneous whole**, CSR (cycle self-recombination) disentangles noise into signal-dependent and independent noises. Zhao, F. et al. (2023).

Allergens were found [...] the chocolate bar and were **homogeneously** distributed [...]. Huet, A.C. et al. (2022).

MEDICAL EDITION

impair (vt) B2

Word family: adj: impaired;
n: impairment (+ n | hearing, speech)

to weaken or damage something, making it less effective or functioning poorly

(vt, adj) + n | ability | effectiveness | performance | function | quality |
+ adv | seriously, severely, significantly, substantially

Dialogue

Patient I've been having trouble with my vision lately.

Doctor If left untreated, these symptoms could **seriously impair** your **ability** / *make it very hard* to perform daily tasks.

Q&A

Questioner Your proposed treatment seems promising, but I have some concerns about potential side effects.

Presenter While all medications carry risks, we've found this approach does not **significantly impair** / *reduce* the **effectiveness** of the treatment in clinical trials.

Informal

Colleague 1 How is that patient who suffered a stroke doing today?

Colleague 2 He seemed confused and had trouble recalling basic information. It could be a sign of **impaired** / *reduced* cognitive **function**. We are running some tests to confirm.

Referral Letter / Discharge Summary

> The patient's chronic pain continues to **impair** / *reduce* her work **performance**, particularly during tasks requiring prolonged standing or walking. This functional **impairment** / *decline* has significantly affected her ability to maintain full-time employment as a retail manager.

Scientific Literature

> Bilateral amygdala lesions **impair** the **ability** to identify certain emotions, especially fear [...]. Atkinson, A.P. et al. (2007)
>
> Brain metastases cause cognitive **impairment** and **impair quality** of life. Shamardani, K., Monje, M. (2023).
>
> Severe congenital **hearing impairment** is an important handicap affecting 0.1% of live-born infants and 1%–2% of graduates of Neonatal Intensive Care Units. Oudesluys-Murphy, A.M. et al. (1996).

imperative (adj)

Word family: n: imperative; adv: imperatively; syn: vital

crucial or urgent; requiring immediate attention or action

+ adj | ethical | +prep | to, that

Dialogue

Patient   I've been having trouble sleeping lately.

Doctor   It's **imperative** / *crucial* **to** identify the underlying cause of your insomnia so it doesn't become a chronic issue.

Q&A

Questioner   Were any ethical considerations taken into account in your study?

Presenter   Ensuring informed consent among participants was an **imperative** / *essential* **step** in conducting ethically sound research.

Informal

Colleague 1   Have you reviewed the latest patient-care guidelines for post-op recovery?

Colleague 2   I have, and they emphasise that early mobility is **imperative** / *essential* **to** reduce the risk of complications like blood clots.

Referral Letter / Discharge Summary

It is **imperative** / *very important* **that** Mrs. Zhang maintains strict glucose monitoring four times daily, given her recent episodes of severe hypoglycemia while alone at home.

Scientific Literature

As unpaid family caregiving of older adults becomes increasingly prevalent, it is **imperative to** understand how family caregivers are socialized and how they understand the caregiving role. McAllum, K. et al. (2021).

It is also **imperative to** note that the SADS-CoV outbreak started in Guangdong province, near the location of the SARS pandemic origin. Dhama, K. et al. (2020).

Transparency in reporting is a fundamental **ethical imperative** of objective scientific research justifying massive official regulations and policies. Aschner, M. et al. (2018).

MEDICAL EDITION

implicit (adj)

Word family: v: imply; n: implication; adv: implicitly; ant: explicit

indirectly suggested or implied rather than stated openly; influencing someone subconsciously or without their awareness

+ prep | in | + n | assumption, bias | message | recognition | suggestion | understanding

Dialogue

Doctor   You haven't said anything outright, but I sense there's an **implicit**/ *hidden* concern **in** what you're asking – what are you worried about?

Patient   I don't want to jump to conclusions, but I researched my symptoms online and I'm worried I might have cancer.

Q&A

Questioner   What is your **implicit assumption** / *presumption* about the control group's baseline characteristics?

Presenter   We assumed that they mirror the general population in our catchment area.

Informal

Colleague 1   There's always that **implicit** / *unspoken* expectation that we'll stay late to finish rounds, even if no one says it outright.

Colleague 2   Tell me about it. I just wish they'd be more upfront instead of assuming we'll read their minds.

Referral Letter / Discharge Summary

The patient's chronic alcohol use poses an **implicit** / *unspoken* (or *inherent*) hepatotoxic risk from the acetaminophen with which he has been self-medicating.

Scientific Literature

Implicit bias appears in multiple facets of medical education, training, and promotion with negative effects on diversity and equity efforts. Ogunleye, T.A. (2023).

The **implicit message** interns hear is to remain silent about insecurities and stress, and, in particular, female students might face disadvantages. Verdonk, P. et al. (2014).

Being able to both place trust in others and decide whether to reciprocate trust placed in us is rooted in **implicit** and explicit processes that guide expectations of others […]. Fareri, D.S. (2019).

incremental (adj)

Word family: n: increment; adj: incrementally

growing gradually in small, consistent amounts

+ n | steps, change | increase, rise | advances, improvements, progress, benefits

Dialogue

Patient I feel like the current medication is not making any difference.

Doctor In that case, we can **incrementally** / *gradually* increase your medication and closely monitor your progress.

Q&A

Questioner Could you discuss the potential applications of these findings in clinical settings?

Presenter Our research suggests an **incremental** / *step-by-step* enhancement in the treatment outcomes.

Informal

Colleague 1 I've recently been checking out different workout classes – would you like to join me one day?

Colleague 2 I'm currently working on my fitness by taking **incremental** / *gradual* steps, such as walking more and using the stairs. Maybe when I'm fitter!

Referral Letter / Discharge Summary

Serial chest radiographs over the past three months have shown **incremental** / *gradual* **advances** in the clearing of her right lower lobe pneumonia, though complete resolution has not yet been achieved.

Scientific Literature

Incremental increases in medication adherence were associated with improved outcomes. Ho, P.M. et al. (2006).

The power of **incremental change** is also behind the Kaizen, a popular business model for industrial engineering first popularized by Toyota […]. Schoppe, K.A. (2017).

'**Incremental benefits** of novel pharmaceuticals in the UK'. Polak, T.B. et al. (2022).

MEDICAL EDITION

induce (vt) `C1`

Word family: n: induction

to prompt or convince someone to take a particular action; to bring about or trigger an effect or condition

---

+ n as object | change | sickness, injury, disease | reaction, response | sleep, coma

Dialogue

Patient I've been feeling nauseous and dizzy since starting the new medication you prescribed.

Doctor The symptoms you're describing suggest that the medication may be **inducing** an adverse **reaction** / *causing side effects*.

Q&A

Questioner I'm curious about the potential side effects that you may have observed during the clinical trial.

Presenter Our data indicates that the drug did not **induce** / *cause* any significant unwanted **changes** in the participants' health status.

Informal

Colleague 1 The swelling in the patient's brain is not going down – do you think we'll need to **induce** / *put him in* a **coma**?

Colleague 2 Probably. It might be the only way to stabilise things and protect the brain.

Referral Letter / Discharge Summary

> The rapidly administered IV fluids **induced** / *caused* a marked improvement in the patient's blood pressure and heart rate.

Scientific Literature

> Ultraviolet-B (UV-B) light plays a crucial role in plant-herbivorous arthropods interactions by **inducing changes** in constitutive and inducible plant defenses. Escobar-Bravo, R. et al. (2017).
>
> Progesterone (P4) is known to **induce** an acrosome **reaction** in mammalian sperm in vitro, whereas cholesterol is a major inhibitor of acrosome reaction. Khorasani, A.M. et al. (2000).
>
> Reported etiologies of coma encountered included medically **induced coma** (24%), traumatic brain injury (24%), intracerebral hemorrhage (21%), and cardiac arrest/hypoxic-ischemic encephalopathy (11%). Helbok, R. et al. (2022).

Application in context

*deduction vs. induction: in research, **deduction** predicts outcomes from general theories, while **induction** derives general conclusions from observed patterns in experiments.*

ENGLISH EXPRESSIONS IN CONTEXT

infer (vt)

Word family: n: inference (v + | draw, make | adj + | causal, logical, reasonable); syn: deduce, conclude

to draw a conclusion based on available evidence or information; to indirectly imply or hint that something is true

adv + | reasonably, correctly, directly

Dialogue

Patient I've been feeling really tired recently and have lost some weight, and I've noticed that I'm always thirsty. Could it be diabetes?

Doctor Based on what I'm hearing, I would **infer** / *think* **that** further tests are necessary to completely rule out diabetes.

Q&A

Questioner Based on your findings, it seems that the participants who followed the exercise routine had a lower incidence of cardiovascular issues – what's your take on that?

Presenter The **inference** / *implication* is that engaging in the exercise routine may lower the probability of cardiovascular issues.

Informal

Colleague 1 These salad greens taste different today.

Colleague 2 Yeah, they've switched suppliers – we can **infer** / *guess* **that** from the change in flavour and packaging.

Referral Letter / Discharge Summary

> Given the acute onset and distribution of the rash, we can **reasonably infer** / *conclude* a diagnosis of herpes zoster.

Scientific Literature

> The recent identification of neural activity with evidence accumulation suggests that it may be possible to **directly infer** what mechanisms vary from an analysis of how neural dynamics vary. Purcell, B.A., Palmeri, T.J. (2017).
>
> It offers a way to **infer** potentially causal relationships between risk factors and outcomes using observational data […]. Levin, M.G., Burgess, S. (2024).
>
> By comparing the outcomes of individuals with different genetic variants, researchers may **draw causal inferences** about the effects of […] disease […]. Levin, M.G., Burgess, S. (2024).

Application in context

> *infer vs. imply: to **infer** is to draw a conclusion from available evidence (done by a listener/reader), while to **imply** is to suggest something indirectly (done by a speaker/writer) – they represent opposite sides of the same communicative process. See page 111.*

MEDICAL EDITION

inherent (adj)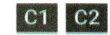

Word family: adv: inherently; syn: intrinsic, inbuilt

a fundamental and permanent characteristic of something or someone that cannot be separated

---

+ n | bias | danger, difficulty | limit, limitation | part | problem | property, quality | risk

Dialogue

Doctor Some of the pain you're feeling may be due to the **inherent** / *specific* **challenges** of your condition – it's not uncommon.

Patient I understand. It's reassuring to know that this is part of the condition and not something unusual happening.

Q&A

Questioner What steps did you take to address the **inherent** / *fundamental* (or *unavoidable*) **problem** of subjective bias in patient-reported outcomes?

Presenter We implemented a double-blind protocol where neither patients nor care providers knew their group assignment.

Informal

Colleague 1 The **inherent** / *usual* noise that comes with living in the city is something can never get used to.

Colleague 2 I totally get that. Even with earplugs, it feels like there's always something going on in the background.

Referral Letter / Discharge Summary

The patient's condition, while not **inherently dangerous** / *dangerous in itself*, requires specialised nephrology follow-up due to the progressive decline in renal function.

Scientific Literature

Rock climbing involves some **inherent danger**, and rock climbers should be able to carry out basic rescue techniques for their own safety. Hawley, A. et al. (2019).

Furthermore, sensitization with formation of anti-drug antibodies is an **inherent limitation** to administration of monoclonal antibodies. Ma, C. et al. (2019).

Frail older people have an **inherent risk** of polypharmacy due to the need to treat multiple comorbidities, thus leading to various negative effects on their health due to the adverse actions from the drugs. Nwadiugwu, M.C. (2020).

integral (adj)

Word family: v: integrate

essential and fundamental to the completeness of a whole; naturally embedded within something rather than external or detachable

+ n | aspect, component, member, part | role | + prep | to

Dialogue

Patient   My knee hurts when I bend it.

Doctor   Regular stretching is **integral to** / *essential for* healing your knee pain.

Q&A

Questioner   How did you account for the potential impact of sleep patterns on your results?

Presenter   Sleep monitoring was an **integral** / *core* **part** of our study design, with daily logs analysed alongside the primary outcomes.

Informal

Colleague 1   Did you hear that Dr. A from Neurology is retiring next month?

Colleague 2   Yes, she's been an **integral** / *key* **member** of our research team for over two decades, and we'll really miss her expertise.

Referral Letter / Discharge Summary

Physical therapy has been an **integral** / *essential* **component** of Mr. J's post-operative care. We recommend that his new care team **integrate** / *incorporate* similar rehabilitation exercises into his ongoing treatment plan.

Scientific Literature

Technological innovation has become an **integral aspect** of our daily life, such as wearable and information technology, virtual reality and the Internet of Things which have contributed to transforming healthcare business and operations. Stoumpos, A.I. et al. (2023).

'It's time to recognize self care as an **integral component** of health systems'. Narasimhan, M. et al. (2019).

MRI is **integral to** the diagnostic work-up of congenital and acquired disorders of the central nervous system in newborns, and [...]. Barkovich, A.J. (2019).

MEDICAL EDITION

interrogate (vt) C2

Word family: n interrogation

to ask intense or aggressive questions over an extended time; to extract data from a machine or system; to question for analysis or deeper understanding

+ n | device (often used for cardiac devices)

Dialogue

Doctor So, I see you've transferred from another doctor's surgery just down the road.

Patient Yes, I didn't like the doctor there. Everytime I went in, I felt like I was being **interrogated** / *questioned* about my lifestyle choices.

Q&A

Questioner Have you looked at other potential factors that could explain the recovery patterns?

Presenter We needed to **interrogate** / *analyse* the age-recovery correlation specifically since our preliminary data showed such unusual patterns.

Informal

Colleague 1 How's the patient with the pacemaker?

Colleague 2 We had to **interrogate** / *access* data from the **device** to check for any issues. It showed some irregularities that might explain the symptoms.

Referral Letter / Discharge Summary

During the psychiatric assessment, the patient exhibited increased anxiety when **interrogated** / *questioned* about his childhood experiences, suggesting possible unresolved trauma. Upon **interrogating** / *examining* the patient's history of recurrent headaches, we found a strong temporal relationship with changes in barometric pressure.

Scientific Literature

In many Western jurisdictions, criminal suspects undergoing police **interrogations** have the right to remain silent. Snow, M.D. et al. (2023).

Recently, the emergence of single-cell RNA sequencing (scRNAseq) has offered a powerful new tool for **interrogating** rheumatic diseases [...]. Zheng, Z. et al. (2022).

Interrogation of tissue informs on patient management through delivery of a diagnosis together with associated clinically relevant data. Ilyas, M. (2017).

intriguing (adj)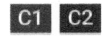

extremely interesting due to being unusual or mysterious

Word family: vt/vi: intrigue; n: intrigue; adj: intrigued; adv: intriguingly

+ n | aspect | example | possibility | question | thought

Dialogue

Patient — Whenever I drink coffee in the morning, I can hear classical music playing from inside my stomach, especially Mozart.

Doctor — How **intriguing** / *fascinating* – I believe what you're experiencing is a rare condition called 'gastric synesthesia' where the caffeine triggers auditory hallucinations synchronised to your digestive movements.

Q&A

Questioner — The most **intriguing** / *remarkable* **aspect** of your research is the correlation between circadian rhythms and autoimmune responses – how did you control for seasonal variations?

Presenter — We used a matched control group from the same geographic region and tracked both groups across a full calendar year.

Informal

Colleague 1 — I've been thinking about how people handle stress differently. It really **intrigues** / *fascinates* **me** how some seem to thrive under pressure.

Colleague 2 — Yeah, it's interesting. I wonder if it's more about personality or if they've learned to cope over time.

Referral Letter / Discharge Summary

After ruling out common autoimmune conditions, the patient's combination of intermittent fever, unusual rash distribution and elevated IL-6 levels raises the **intriguing** / *unusual* **possibility** of an adult-onset autoinflammatory syndrome requiring rheumatology consultation.

Scientific Literature

Overall, our results represent an **intriguing example** of killing bacteria by activating a non-essential enzyme, and thus expand the scope of antibiotic targets beyond the traditional essential proteins or pathways. Cho, H. et al. (2020).

The dual functions of TMEM16F as Ca(2+)-activated ion channel and lipid scramblase raise **intriguing questions** regarding their molecular basis. Feng, S. et al. (2023).

Intriguingly, multiple types of sleep have recently been found in animals ranging from non-avian reptiles to arthropods to cephalopods. Rattenborg, N.C., Ungurean, G. (2022).

MEDICAL EDITION

intrinsic (adj) `C2`

Word family: adv: intrinsically; ant: extrinsic

essential and inherent to the true nature of something or someone

+ n | character, motivation, characteristic | factor | nature, property, quality | part | meaning | value

Dialogue

Doctor — Finding **intrinsic** / *self-motivated* **motivation** to stick with your therapy is really important for long-term recovery.

Patient — I see what you mean. When I'm motivated for my own good, it feels easier to stay committed, rather than just doing it because I'm told to.

Q&A

Questioner — How does your research address the **intrinsic** / *personal* **nature** of pain perception to vary from patient to patient?

Presenter — We developed a personalised baseline-measurement protocol that calibrates each individual's pain scale before starting the treatment.

Informal

Colleague 1 — It's been a real challenge to get undergrad students engaged in biostats lectures.

Colleague 2 — Well, making the students solve real clinical case studies during class has become an **intrinsic** / *essential* **part** of my teaching approach. Perhaps you could give that a go?

Referral Letter / Discharge Summary

The patient's ventricular tachycardia appears to be **intrinsically** / *directly* **linked** to her abnormal electrolyte levels, particularly the persistent hypokalemia.

Scientific Literature

Increasing evidence, both functional and morphological, supports the concept of increased intestinal permeability as an **intrinsic characteristic** of type 1 diabetes (T1D) in both humans and animal models of the disease. Li, X., Atkinson, M.A. (2015).

Available evidence is limited to short-term effects on clinical rating scales which may be difficult to interpret and have limited **intrinsic meaning** to patients. Jönsson, L. et al. (2024).

Intrinsic factor (IF)* was first identified as a component of the gastric mucosa that reacted with an extrinsic factor, later discovered to be vitamin B12 (VB12). Alpers, D.H., Russell-Jones, G. (2013).

invoke (vt) `C1`

Word family: n: invocation

to cite a law or principle as justification for action; to reference a person, concept or example to strengthen an argument or explain a decision

+ n as object | **authority** | **name** | **principle** | **right**

Dialogue

Patient I'd like to **invoke** / *exercise* my **right** to a second opinion before proceeding with the suggested treatment.

Doctor Of course, that's your prerogative, and I can provide you with a list of qualified specialists in this field for consultation.

Q&A

Questioner Regarding end-of-life decisions, how can we **invoke** / *apply* the **principle** of patient autonomy while ensuring we're not abandoning our duty of care?

Presenter The reality is that there is no easy answer to that question.

Informal

Colleague 1 I think we should relax the dress-code policy and allow jeans in the office every day, not just on Fridays.

Colleague 2 That's an interesting suggestion, but management might **invoke** / *cite* the professional-image clause in our company policy to resist such a change.

Referral Letter / Discharge Summary

After exhausting standard treatments, Dr. Roberts **invoked** / *used* her clinical discretion to pursue an experimental therapy regimen.

Scientific Literature

Efforts to explain animal population cycles often **invoke** consumer-resource **theory**, which has shown that consumer-resource interactions alone can drive population cycles. Dwyer, G. et al. (2022).

Psychology, including health psychology, frequently **invokes** the concept of belief but almost never defines it. Cromby, J. (2012).

MEDICAL EDITION

manifest (vt, vi, adj) C1

Word family: n: manifestation

to display or exhibit something clearly, particularly emotions or traits; to emerge or become apparent; (adj) obvious or readily perceived

+ n | disease, symptom | + adv | clinically

Dialogue

Patient I've been having trouble smelling and tasting things lately, and my throat feels scratchy.

Doctor These **symptoms** can **manifest** / *appear* following a COVID-19 infection, particularly affecting your ENT* system.

Q&A

Questioner What did you observe in your study as **manifest** / *obvious* **symptoms**?

Presenter We observed fatigue, joint pain and cognitive difficulties as the most common **manifest** / *visible* **symptoms** across our patient cohort.

Informal

Colleague 1 Hey, did you see the latest data from the clinical trials?

Colleague 2 Yeah, I was surprised by the unexpected **manifestation** / *appearance* of neurological symptoms in what we thought was primarily a cardiovascular issue.

Referral Letter / Discharge Summary

The patient's condition initially **manifested** / *showed up* as a cluster of non-specific symptoms, including fatigue, mild fever and generalised body aches.

Scientific Literature

In dermatology, **diseases** that **manifest** as blisters or blister-like lesions are common […]. Hu, Y. (2019).

Studies suggest **clinically manifest** cardiac involvement occurs in 5% of patients with pulmonary/systemic sarcoidosis. Birnie, D. et al. (2015).

The Parkinson's disease (PD) research field has seen the advent of several promising biomarkers and a deeper understanding of the clinical features of the disease from the earliest stages of pathology to **manifest disease**. Chahine, L.M. et al. (2023).

ENGLISH EXPRESSIONS IN CONTEXT

mitigate (vt)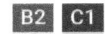

Word family: n: mitigation

to reduce the severity, intensity or negative effects of something undesirable; to lessen the impact of a harmful or difficult situation

(vt) + n as object | **effect, impact** | **issue, problem, risk, severity** | **suffering** | **damage, harm** | **consequences** | **stress, symptom** | (adj) + n | **strategy**

Dialogue

Patient I've been experiencing persistent back pain and numbness in my legs lately.

Doctor We need to diagnose the underlying cause and determine the best course of treatment to **mitigate** / *reduce* the **severity** of your symptoms.

Q&A

Questioner Given the potential side effects of the proposed treatment, have you considered any alternative approaches?

Presenter Yes, we've developed a comprehensive **mitigation** / *risk-reduction* **strategy** that includes careful patient monitoring and dose adjustments to minimise risks while maintaining therapeutic efficacy.

Informal

Colleague 1 Did you hear about the new project-management software the university is planning to implement?

Colleague 2 I've been looking into it, and it seems like it could really help **mitigate** / *reduce* some of the scheduling **issues** we've been having with our current system.

Referral Letter / Discharge Summary

We initiated oral prokinetics to **mitigate** / *ease* her abdominal **symptoms**. This **mitigation** / *relief* approach has reduced her daily pain episodes by half.

Scientific Literature

Exercise may not **mitigate** the ill **effects** of prolonged sitting. Kennedy, M.S. (2018).

The impact of rising temperatures on livestock in Egypt was reviewed, where extensive resources to **mitigate** the **impact** are not often available. Goma, A.A., Phillips, C.J.C. (2022).

This article attempts to identify the most pressing roadblocks in patient recruitment, categorizes them based on the stakeholders involved and provides suggestions on how to identify and **mitigate** the **risks** involved. Bogin, V. (2022).

A key disease **mitigation strategy** is vector control, which relies heavily on the use of insecticides. Conway, M.J. et al. (2023).

MEDICAL EDITION

mundane (adj)

Word family: n: mundaneness; adv: mundanely;
syn: unremarkable, dull

ordinary and dull, lacking excitement or interest

+ n | task | aspect | detail

Dialogue

Patient Sometimes, I feel like my life is stuck in a **mundane** / *dull* routine, and I don't know how to break free from it.

Doctor It's common to feel that way, but identifying small changes can help bring new energy and purpose into your daily life.

Q&A

Questioner Thank you for the informative presentation – can you elaborate on the potential side effects of this new treatment?

Presenter While the treatment shows promise, we must thoroughly assess any potential side effects, even those that might seem **mundane** / *common*, to ensure patient safety and efficacy.

Informal

Colleague 1 Did you catch the keynote speaker's presentation this morning? It was quite insightful.

Colleague 2 Yes, I did. While some topics were familiar, others provided fresh perspectives, making it far from **mundane** / *ordinary*.

Referral Letter / Discharge Summary

The patient's recovery from appendectomy has followed a **mundane** / *routine* course, with appropriate wound-healing and no post-operative complications noted.

Scientific Literature

Obtaining informed consent has been traditionally viewed as a **mundane task**, learned on the job and often relegated [...]. Anandaiah, A., Rock, L. (2019).

Complications of endoscopic sinus surgery (ESS) can range from the **mundane** to the catastrophic, with nasal hemorrhage being the most common. Humphreys, I.M., Hwang, P.H. (2015).

They craft stories of carrying (in)visible labor, isolation, simultaneity, and list-keeping as they navigate the **mundaneness** of everyday pandemic home/work/life. Guyotte, K.W. et al. (2023).

Application in context

*mundane vs. mediocre: while **mundane** describes something ordinary or routine without judgment, **mediocre** specifically implies disappointing or below-average quality.*

ENGLISH EXPRESSIONS IN CONTEXT

myriad (n, adj) C1

(n) a vast, uncountable multitude of things; (adj) very large quantity

(adj) + n | options, ways | variety | other | (n) + prep | of

Dialogue

Patient My stomach has been hurting for three days and I wonder why.

Doctor There's a **myriad of** / *many* possible explanations. Abdominal pain requires a thorough examination to diagnose the issue.

Q&A

Questioner How does your research address the gap in current treatment protocols?

Presenter The **myriad of** / *numerous* factors we uncovered through our clinical trials suggests a complete overhaul of existing therapeutic approaches.

Informal

Colleague 1 Did you hear they're planning to convert the old break room into a meditation space?

Colleague 2 Yeah, but I'd rather they fixed the parking situation first and addressed the **myriad** / *countless* **other** infrastructure problems in this building.

Referral Letter / Discharge Summary

Despite the patient's chronic heart condition affecting her health in **myriad** / *many different* **ways**, she has maintained remarkable adherence to her medication regimen and lifestyle modifications.

Scientific Literature

Here I discuss my motivations and their impact on how I conduct my research as one example of the **myriad ways** to be a scientist. Serio, T.R. (2016).

A **myriad variety** of therapeutic agents or chemical substances can induce either a transient or persistent increase in blood pressure, or interfere with the blood pressure-lowering effects of antihypertensive drugs. Grossman, E., Messerli, F.H. (2012).

This review critically evaluates the latest literature that supports the **myriad** treatment **options** for infantile hemangiomas. Keller, R.G., Patel, K.G. (2015).

The human body is populated by **myriads of** microorganisms throughout its surface and in the cavities connected to the outside. Alvarez, J. et al. (2021).

MEDICAL EDITION

perceive (vt)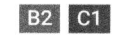

Word family: n: perception; syn: see

to view or interpret someone/something in a specific way; to notice or become aware of something

+ n as object | danger | pain | difference | reality, world |
adv + | commonly, generally, widely

Dialogue

Patient I've noticed that when I'm stressed, the pain seems to intensify.

Doctor **Pain** is actually **perceived** / *registered* in the brain, so sometimes there's a mental element to it – stress or anxiety can make it feel worse.

Q&A

Questioner How did your team achieve such remarkable outcomes with this challenging patient population?

Presenter Our data suggests that this therapeutic approach is far more effective than **commonly perceived** / *most people think*.

Informal

Colleague 1 It's interesting how different people **perceive** / *experience* the side effects of the same medication. Some have mild reactions, while others feel much worse.

Colleague 2 Yeah, it's all about individual sensitivity. The way our bodies process the drug can vary so much.

Referral Letter / Discharge Summary

The elderly patient's altered **perception** / *awareness* of time and place during evening hours suggests an evolving sundown syndrome* that warrants geriatric consultation.

Scientific Literature

Traits of 'negativity bias' reflect the tendency to **perceive danger** rather than reward related information [...]. Williams, L.M. et al. (2015).

The idea that predictions shape how we **perceive** and comprehend the **world** has become increasingly influential in the field of systems neuroscience. Teufel, C., Fletcher, P.C. (2020).

True lactose intolerance (symptoms stemming from lactose malabsorption) is less common than is **widely perceived**, and should be viewed as just one potential cause of cows' milk intolerance. Pal, S. et al. (2015).

ENGLISH EXPRESSIONS IN CONTEXT

postulate (vt, vi)

Word family: n: postulation, postulate; syn: posit

to propose something as true or factual to serve as a foundation for developing theories or further ideas

+ n | existence

Dialogue

Patient I've had this terrible burning sensation in my chest for the past three days, especially after eating spicy foods.

Doctor Based on your symptoms, I **postulate** / *believe* **that** you're suffering from acid reflux.

Q&A

Questioner Your **postulate** / *theory* that chronic inflammation directly triggers genetic mutations seems to contradict conventional knowledge.

Presenter While I understand your concern, our findings actually complement data from other studies.

Informal

Colleague 1 Sometimes I wonder if consciousness is really just an illusion created by our brains to make sense of reality.

Colleague 2 I am more inclined to **postulate** the **existence** of / *believe in* a fundamental consciousness field that permeates the universe.

Referral Letter / Discharge Summary

We **postulate** / *believe* **that** the patient's recurrent episodes of syncope are cardiogenic in origin, based on the characteristic ECG changes during these events. This **postulation** / *conclusion* is further supported by the positive tilt table test and the family history of long QT syndrome.

Scientific Literature

We **postulate that** endocrinology care will be completely reinvented in the Digital Age. Dalan, R. et al. (2022).

The initial **postulated** mechanisms for development of post-traumatic pseudolipomas were anatomically and mechanically based. Galea, L.A. et al. (2009).

Indeed, a substantial body of evidence has meanwhile been accumulated in favour of this **postulate**. Eiden, M. et al. (2006).

Application in context

postulate vs. posit: **postulate** *implies a formal foundational assumption in scientific contexts, whereas* **posit** *represents a straightforward proposition of ideas.*

MEDICAL EDITION

potent (adj)

 Word family: n: potency; adv: potently; ant: impotent (lacking power), powerless; syn: powerful

having a powerful impact on the body or mind; extremely intense, forceful or powerful

+ n | antidote* | combination, compound | effect | force | inhibitor | mix, mixture

Dialogue

Patient — While hiking yesterday, I was bitten by what I think was a coral snake.

Doctor — Don't worry, I have a **potent antidote** / *effective treatment* that will neutralise the venom.

Q&A

Questioner — How does the combination of compounds A and B achieve such remarkable efficacy?

Presenter — The **potent** / *powerful* **mixture** works by simultaneously disrupting the bacterial cell wall and inhibiting protein synthesis.

Informal

Colleague 1 — Did you see how our new research collaboration with the physics department is revolutionising medical imaging?

Colleague 2 — Yes, cross-disciplinary innovation is a **potent** / *driving* **force** in advancing healthcare technology.

Referral Letter / Discharge Summary

The patient was prescribed **increasingly potent** / *progressively stronger* opioid analgesics during the final weeks of palliative care to maintain adequate pain control.

Scientific Literature

Acetylcholine is a **potent** excitatory neurotransmitter, crucial for cognition and the control of alertness and arousal. Platt, B., Riedel, G. (2011).

Using a drug discovery scheme for Alzheimer's disease (AD) that is based upon multiple pathologies of old age, we identified a **potent compound** with efficacy in rodent memory and AD animal models. Chiruta, C. et al. (2013).

Cytokines and cytokine receptor antagonist showed **potent effect** of alleviating the development of morphine tolerance. Liu, D.Q. et al. (2019).

The **potencies** of topical corticosteroid products have mainly been classified using clinical data but [...]. Zvidzayi, M. et al. (2021).

ENGLISH EXPRESSIONS IN CONTEXT

premise (n, vt) C1

Word family: adj: premised; syn: assumption

a foundational idea or belief that supports a conclusion or guides action; (vt) to establish an argument or concept on a particular assumption or basis

+ prep | **of** | sub conj + | **that** | exp | **on/upon the premise that**

Dialogue

Patient   I feel a sharp pain behind my kneecap whenever I walk up stairs.

Doctor   **On the premise that** / *Since* your pain only occurs with climbing motions, I suspect it might be patellofemoral syndrome.

Q&A

Questioner   I challenge the **premise** / *grounds* **of** your statistical analysis, as your sample size appears too small to draw such broad conclusions.

Presenter   I acknowledge your concern, but our power calculations indicated that the sample size was sufficient.

Informal

Colleague 1   I'm thinking of switching our lab meetings from Monday mornings to Friday afternoons to boost attendance.

Colleague 2   The **premise** / *idea* **that** people are more likely to engage on Fridays doesn't match my experience in academic settings.

Referral Letter / Discharge Summary

While the initial **premise of** our diagnostic workup was a suspected paraneoplastic syndrome, the patient's subsequent course and negative extensive malignancy screening have led us to revise our working diagnosis.

Scientific Literature

It is quite evident that when the **premises** are wrong or too vague the unavoidable consequences will be a negative outcome. Gattinoni, L. et al. (2015).

Biologists and psychologists are re-thinking the long-standing **premise of** genes as the primary cause of development [...]. Lickliter, R. (2017).

It is **upon** this **premise that** all the observations put forth in this study are centred [...]. Contini, P., Osmanaj, E. (2023).

However, much of this existing evidence requires a new look, because it is **premised on** a fundamental ambiguity. Goodwin, G.P., Gromet, D.M. (2014).

MEDICAL EDITION

proliferate (vi) C1

Word family: n: proliferation syn: multiply

to multiply or increase rapidly in amount or number

+ n | cell

Dialogue

Patient My gums bleed when I brush my teeth.

Doctor Poor oral hygiene allows bacteria to **proliferate** / *multiply* between your teeth and gums.

Q&A

Questioner Given that cancer **cells proliferate** / *grow* more rapidly in acidic environments, have you considered measuring the pH levels in your experimental model?

Presenter Yes, we monitored pH throughout the study.

Informal

Colleague 1 I heard you're planning to buy that house near the botanical garden.

Colleague 2 Yes, but I'm worried by the way the ivy **proliferates** / *spreads* and could damage the brickwork on the walls.

Referral Letter / Discharge Summary

The patient's abnormal skin **cells** continue to **proliferate** / *multiply* despite the initial course of topical steroids. Skin biopsy revealed increased **cellular proliferation** / *cell growth* with atypical morphology, suggesting the need for further immunohistochemical analysis.

Scientific Literature

Lymphoid tissue analogous to gut mucosa-associated lymphoid tissue **proliferates** in the skin in response to antigenic stimulation. Hussein, M.R. (2013).

In both young and elderly women, all NK subsets **proliferated** and died more rapidly than T cells. Lutz, C.T. et al. (2011).

However, it remains unclear whether microglia **proliferate** in the affected area, and the mechanism of the **proliferation** has long attracted the attention of researchers. Ishijima, T., Nakajima, K. (2023).

ENGLISH EXPRESSIONS IN CONTEXT

prove (vt)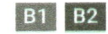

Word family: n: proof; ant: disprove

to demonstrate the truth of something using facts or evidence; (linking verb) to become known as having a particular quality over time

+ n | theory | + adv | otherwise | + adj | true, false

Dialogue

Patient Is it true that my test results show clear **proof** / *signs* of an underlying issue?

Doctor I'm afraid that your test results strongly indicate an underlying issue in your abdomen.

Q&A

Questioner How certain are you that the observed changes are due solely to the intervention and not influenced by other variables?

Presenter The observed changes are consistent across controlled conditions, suggesting that the intervention constitutes compelling **proof** / *evidence* of its impact.

Informal

Colleague 1 Those rumours about elephants having exceptional memory have been **proven** to be **true** / *correct* through recent cognitive studies.

Colleague 2 Makes sense, since their temporal lobes are way larger than ours.

Referral Letter / Discharge Summary

The patient improved on a conservative management plan until cultures **proved otherwise** / *showed different results*, necessitating a switch to broad-spectrum antibiotics.

Scientific Literature

There is a huge increase in stories on social media that may initially appear credible but later **prove false** or fabricated [...]. Naeem, B.S., Bhatti, R. (2020).

Although the sighting of a single black swan suffices to **disprove** the **theory** that all swans are white, sceptics may argue that the light was poor and that the swan looked grey. Gorchein, A. (1997).

This was confirmed in a **proof-of-concept** study in patients with nontransfusion-dependent thalassemias. Matte, A. et al. (2023).

Application in context

proof vs. evidence: **proof** *definitively demonstrates truth, while* **evidence** *merely suggests or supports it. See page 112.*

In academic/research settings, **prove** *(and its noun form* **proof***) are often collocated with words that are related to theory or logic.*

provoke (vt)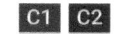

Word family: n: provocation; adj: provocative

to deliberately trigger a specific response or outcome; to intentionally annoy or upset someone, causing an angry response

+ n as object | argument, attack, controversy, criticism, debate, discussion | reaction, response | thought | exp | thought-provoking

Dialogue

Patient My chest hurts when I drink coffee.

Doctor Caffeine can **provoke** / *cause* irregular heartbeats.

Q&A

Questioner Your findings about diet and cancer survival may **provoke controversy** / *cause disagreement* among oncologists.

Presenter That is possible, but our findings are based on high-quality longitudinal data from a large cohort.

Informal

Colleague 1 Have you seen the research showing that gut bacteria might influence our food cravings?

Colleague 2 That study is certainly **thought-provoking** / *makes me think*. Microbial communities could apparently be manipulating our behaviour.

Referral Letter / Discharge Summary

Exercise seems to reliably **provoke** / *cause* chest discomfort. During treadmill testing, symptoms appeared at six minutes of moderate exertion without any additional **provocation** / *trigger*.

Scientific Literature

But precisely how tissues are transformed continues to **provoke controversy** and **debate**, hindering cancer prevention and early intervention strategies. Jassim, A. et al. (2023).

However, it is uncertain whether the minute amounts remaining could **provoke** allergic **reactions** in highly susceptible individuals. Crevel, R.W. et al. (2000).

Scientific effort over the last 5 years has focused on precise evaluation of the stimuli that **provoke sickness** and on the development of behavioural and new pharmacological interventions to suppress sickness. Golding, J.F., Gresty, M.A. (2005).

ENGLISH EXPRESSIONS IN CONTEXT

ramp up (phrV)

Word family: n: ramp-up; ant: ramp down

to intensify, accelerate, or boost something's quantity, scale or pace

+ n as object | production | phase | efforts | dosage | dose

Dialogue

Patient The pharmacist mentioned something about gradually increasing my dosage. Can you explain that?

Doctor Of course. For this medication, we use a four-week **dose ramp-up** / *gradual increase*. So, we'll start with a lower dose and gradually increase it each week until you reach the full amount. This will help your body adjust and reduces the risk of side effects.

Q&A

Questioner How close are we to applying nanotechnology to targeted cancer treatment?

Presenter While we've made significant progress in the development of nanoparticle-based cancer therapies, there's still a need to **ramp up** / *increase* our **efforts** on various fronts, such as clinical trials and regulatory approval processes.

Informal

Colleague 1 How's your new project involving AI-assisted diagnosis of rare genetic disorders going?

Colleague 2 We still need to **ramp up** / *improve* our data collection efforts to train the AI model effectively.

Referral Letter / Discharge Summary

Following clinical stabilisation, we have begun to **ramp up** / *gradually increase* his antidepressant **dosage** according to the recommended titration schedule.

Scientific Literature

Can collaborative robots **ramp up** the **production** of medical ventilators? Malik, A.A. et al. (2020).

In the experimental groups, patients received daily venetoclax (400 mg orally) for ten cycles after a 5-week **ramp-up phase** starting on day 22 of cycle 1. Fürstenau, M. et al. (2024).

Some of us may recall a time in healthcare when it seemed that the summer months were a bit quieter, providing an opportunity to catch our breath before the onslaught of fall and the **ramp-up** to flu season. Wojtak, A., Suart, N. (2023).

MEDICAL EDITION

regimen (n) C1

Word family: syn: regime

a structured plan of diet, exercise or medical treatment aimed at maintaining or improving health

adj + | strict | daily | dietary, drug, food | exercise, training | antibiotic, chemotherapy, treatment |
v + | follow | maintain | use

Dialogue

Patient   The rash hasn't improved at all since my last visit.

Doctor   Are you following the **treatment regimen** / *plan* exactly as prescribed, including applying the cream three times daily?

Q&A

Questioner   What's the mechanism behind the observed resistance to your treatment?

Presenter   We maintain this **regimen** / *protocol* to understand the epigenetic modifications in response cells.

Informal

Colleague 1   Did you notice that Dr. Z looks so energetic lately despite his crazy surgery schedule?

Colleague 2   Yeah, he's been following an **exercise regimen** / *routine* that combines sprint intervals and yoga before rounds.

Referral Letter / Discharge Summary

> The patient should continue to follow the **antibiotic regimen** / *schedule* of oral amoxicillin 500mg three times daily for seven more days.

Scientific Literature

> The current front-line **treatment regimen** for drug-sensitive (DS) M. tb* strains is a 6-month protocol involving four different drugs that [...]. Alsayed, S.S.R., Gunosewaya, H. (2023).
>
> Energy-restricted diet is a specific **dietary regimen**, including the continuous energy-restricted diet and the intermittent energy-restricted diet. Zhang, B. et al. (2023).
>
> Older children and adolescents often relax the diet and at some age become reluctant to stick to a **strict regimen**. van Spronsen, F.J., et al. (2017).

ENGLISH EXPRESSIONS IN CONTEXT

remit (vt, vi) `C1`

Word family: n: remission, remittance; remit

(medical) to decrease in intensity or abate (of symptoms/disease); (common usage) to transfer or send money or payment to someone

adv + vi | partially, completely | spontaneously | temporarily |
exp | within someone's remit

Dialogue

Patient   I hope my back symptoms won't come back.

Doctor   We'll closely monitor your condition to ensure this isn't just a **temporary remission** / *brief period of improvement*.

Q&A

Questioner   Given your findings, what policy changes do you think should be implemented to address this issue?

Presenter   That's an important consideration, but recommending policy changes is not **within my remit** / *area of expertise*.

Informal

Colleague 1   Did you get the **remittance** / *payment* details from the patient's insurer?

Colleague 2   No, but I'll follow up again today.

Referral Letter / Discharge Summary

> The patient's nausea and vomiting **completely remitted** / *stopped entirely* after three days of intravenous infusion.

Scientific Literature

> He subsequently developed increasing pain of the left chest wall that did not **remit**, which prevented him from performing manual labor. Foel, O.F. et al. (2020).

> Overall, all patients had either **partially** or **completely remitted**, with none of the patients left with nephrotic range proteinuria. Kumar, S. et al. (2012).

Application in context

> **remit** *as a verb has two noun forms (remission and remittance). In British English,* **remit** *is also used as a noun. See page 112.*

MEDICAL EDITION

resolve (vt, vi)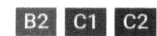

Word family: n: resolution, resolve; syn: settle

to solve a problem; to firmly decide on taking a specific course of action; to make a definite decision to do something

+ n as object | **conflict, controversy, debate** | **difference, disagreement, dispute** | **issue, matter, problem, question, situation** | **uncertainty**

Dialogue

Patient   I want to keep smoking. I don't think it affects my lungs.

Doctor   Let's **resolve** / *settle* this **difference** of opinion by reviewing your latest chest X-rays.

Q&A

Questioner   Your data seems to contradict the Anderson study from last year.

Presenter   Let me **resolve** / *clear up* this **issue** by showing how our different patient populations led to divergent outcomes.

Informal

Colleague 1   I heard a rumour that the cafeteria will replace our favourite coffee machine with a vending machine.

Colleague 2   I'm tired of this speculation. Let me **resolve** this **matter** / *find out* by checking with the facilities manager.

Referral Letter / Discharge Summary

We will continue to monitor the patient's response to the adjusted medication regimen and aim to **resolve** / *fix* this **situation** before considering surgical intervention.

Scientific Literature

Previous explanatory reasoning research shows that people construct causal explanations to **resolve** causal **conflicts**. Kelly, L.J., Khemlani, S. (2023).

The decision-making process and factors influencing parents' decision, how to **resolve disagreement**, what treatment can be withheld or withdrawn are explained. Aladangady, N., de Rooy, L. (2012).

Methodical testing of the multiple potential factors influencing immune responses, as well as refined quantitative methodologies to facilitate optimal dosing strategies, could help **resolve uncertainty** of therapeutic approaches. Shemesh, C.S. et al. (2021).

robust (adj)

Word family: n: robustness; adv: robustly

physically strong and vigorous; durable and resilient to frequent use; (of a system or organisation) resilient and unlikely to collapse or weaken

+ n | evidence | design, methodology | findings, results | nature | immune system | + prep | to, in

Dialogue

Patient How confident are you that this new treatment will work for me?

Doctor The clinical trials provide **robust** / *strong* **evidence** of its effectiveness, so I'm optimistic it'll benefit you too.

Q&A

Questioner How can we be sure that the findings from this research are reliable and applicable to a broad population?

Presenter The research **methodology** employed in our study was **robust** / *rigorous*, incorporating diverse participants and stringent controls to ensure the validity and generalisability of our results.

Informal

Colleague 1 Any recommendations for a good book to read?

Colleague 2 Absolutely, I just finished this novel – it has a **robust** / *strong* plot with intriguing characters that you will enjoy.

Referral Letter / Discharge Summary

The patient's **robust** / *strong* **immune system** and excellent response to the initial antibiotic regimen suggest a favourable prognosis, though continued monitoring is recommended.

Scientific Literature

Robust evidence is essential for policymakers commissioning peer support and practitioners delivering services in health care and community settings. Price, A. et al. (2022).

Strengths of this trial include its **robust design** and high completion rate. Loomba, R. et al. (2023).

Sample sizes were large (1,818 exposed in case-control and 16,824 in cohort studies), providing relatively **robust findings**. Einarson, T.R. et al. (2012).

There have been repeated observations that proteins are surprisingly **robust to** site mutations, enduring significant numbers of substitutions with little change in structure, stability, or function. Taverna, D.M., Goldstein, R.A. (2002).

MEDICAL EDITION

sentient (adj) `C1`

Word family: n: sentience

capable of perceiving through senses or experiencing feelings

+ n | being

Dialogue

Patient   Doctor, I'm worried about being put under anaesthesia for my upcoming surgery.

Doctor   I understand your concern, but rest assured that even while unconscious, you remain a **sentient being** / *thinking, feeling person*, and our entire medical team is committed to your well-being throughout the procedure.

Q&A

Questioner   Given the rapid advancements in AI, do you foresee a future where machines might achieve **sentience** / *consciousness* and potentially replace human healthcare providers?

Presenter   While AI will undoubtedly enhance healthcare delivery, the uniquely human aspects of empathy, intuition and complex decision-making will remain essential in patient care for the foreseeable future.

Informal

Colleague 1   Did you hear about the case in the ICU last night?

Colleague 2   Yes! The patient regained consciousness after days in a coma. But it'll take more time to assess whether they've regained full **sentience** / *ability to feel sensations*, you know?

Note

> The word 'sentient' is rarely used in patient documentation since medical professionals typically use more specific clinical terms to describe a patient's level of consciousness or mental status. You'd more likely see something like: "Patient is alert and oriented to person, place and time." or "Patient demonstrates appropriate level of consciousness and responds to verbal commands."

Scientific Literature

> Decapod crustaceans (crabs, hermit crabs, lobsters, crayfish, shrimps, prawns) are **sentient beings**, not only responding to noxious stimuli but also being capable of feeling pain, discomfort, and distress. De Souza Valente, C. (2022).

> It rests on the notion of a generative model as underwriting (i) **sentient** processing in the brain, and (ii) the scientific process in psychiatry. Friston, K. (2023).

Application in context

> *conscious vs. sentient:* **conscious** *refers to being aware and responsive to surroundings, while* **sentient** *emphasises the ability to feel sensations.*

ENGLISH EXPRESSIONS IN CONTEXT

speculate (vt, vi)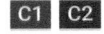

Word family: n: speculation; adj: speculative

to form a belief or assumption without complete information; to invest in assets like property or stocks, hoping for profit while accepting potential loss

+ prep | about | as to | on, upon | sub conj + | that

Dialogue

Patient My stomach has been hurting for three weeks.

Doctor At this stage, I can only **speculate as to** / *guess* the cause. Let's run some tests.

Q&A

Questioner Why do you think these specific tumour cells are more resistant to chemotherapy?

Presenter We **speculate** / *guess* **that** the enhanced membrane proteins block drug absorption, but we need more experiments to confirm this mechanism.

Informal

Colleague 1 Have you heard about the new biotech startup? They're developing a pretty innovative treatment.

Colleague 2 Yeah, I'm tempted to **speculate on** / *invest in* their shares, but it's pretty risky. The returns could be huge, but so could the losses.

Referral Letter / Discharge Summary

The aetiology of her recurrent abdominal pain remains **speculative** / *unclear* despite extensive workup. In light of this diagnostic **speculation** / *uncertainty*, we recommend referral to a tertiary gastroenterology centre for further evaluation.

Scientific Literature

Natural histories map sameness and difference rather than **speculate about** causes. Zachar, P., Kendler, K.S. (2017).

This article outlines these findings and **speculates on** the consequences of the resultant firing symmetries and asymmetries for spatial coding and cognition. Jeffery, K.J. (2023).

One may **speculate that** asthmatics are more sensitive to irritants in the air than healthy subjects […]. Johanson, G. (2020).

Several classifications and definition were made until now and **speculations** still exist on its etiology. As the etiology remains **speculative** the treatment models remain in discussion also. Magnan, J. et al. (2018).

MEDICAL EDITION

stagnate (vi) B2

Word family: n: stagnation; adj: stagnant

to cease development or advancement; to remain motionless without growth; (adj) not flowing or moving, often causing an unpleasant smell

adj + | **stagnant** | + n | economy | water, pond

Dialogue

Patient   I started feeling better but recently I've gone back to feeling really tired and unmotivated.

Doctor   It sounds like your mental health might be **stagnating** / *is not improving* – let's discuss some strategies to help you move forward.

Q&A

Questioner   How do you advise dealing with the recent **stagnation** / *lack of growth* in funding for rare-disease research?

Presenter   I believe we can leverage collaborative networks and emerging technologies to continue making progress in rare-disease research, despite funding challenges.

Informal

Colleague 1   Have you noticed how the local park's **pond** has become really **stagnant** / *motionless* lately?

Colleague 2   Yeah, it's a shame – we should talk to the city about implementing some aeration systems to improve the water quality.

Referral Letter / Discharge Summary

> Despite aggressive fluid management, the patient's renal function continued to **stagnate** / *show no improvement*, necessitating a nephrology consultation.

Scientific Literature

> As maternal mortality and morbidity rates **stagnate** or increase worldwide, there is an urgent need to address health system issues that impede access to high-quality care. Karp, C. et al. (2024).
>
> The probabilities of death **stagnate** between 110 and 115 years, and all the computed probabilities fall below the ceiling of 0.6. Robine, J., Vaupel, J.W. (2001).
>
> Results from longitudinal studies show a **stagnant** or declining rate of epilepsy surgery over time […]. Jetté, N. et al. (2016).

strenuous (adj)

Word family: n: strenuousness; adv: strenuously; syn: arduous

demanding significant effort and physical exertion; characterised by strong determination and vigorous energy

+ n as object | **activity, effort, exercise, exertion, training**

Dialogue

Patient I've been feeling exhausted after my workouts lately.

Doctor It's possible the **exercises** you're doing are too **strenuous** / *intense* – try reducing the intensity to see if it helps.

Q&A

Questioner What are the recommended guidelines for patients recovering from heart surgery regarding **strenuous** / *intense* physical **activity**?

Presenter Post-operative patients should gradually increase their exercise routine, starting with low-impact activities and avoiding **strenuous exertion** / *hard effort* for at least six weeks.

Informal

Colleague 1 I've been training for a marathon, and the **strenuous** / *sustained* **training** has been really challenging.

Colleague 2 It's impressive that you've committed to such an intensive programme.

Referral Letter / Discharge Summary

The patient made **strenuous** / *intense* **efforts** during each physical therapy session, **strenuously** / *vigorously* working to regain function in her affected limb.

Scientific Literature

There is some evidence that **strenuous exercise** may cause and worsen pelvic organ prolapse, but data are inconsistent. Bø, K., Nygaard, I.E. (2020).

Despite the **strenuous effort** to find a suitable treatment option for these amyloid disorders, very few compounds had made it to unsuccessful clinical trials. Low, K.J.Y. et al. (2021).

This paper examines the relationship between the physical **strenuousness** of work and the BMI in Finland […]. Böckerman, P. et al. (2008).

MEDICAL EDITION

succumb (vi) `C2`

Word family: n: succumbence (rarely used)

to be unable to resist an attack, temptation, or pressure; to die as a result of illness or injury

+ prep | **to**

Dialogue

Patient I've been feeling really short of breath lately, even after minimal activity.

Doctor Given your medical history, I'm concerned you may **succumb to** / *fall victim to* heart failure if we don't intervene promptly with treatment.

Q&A

Questioner Won't all patients eventually **succumb to** / *die from* this disease regardless of the treatment you propose?

Presenter While our treatment cannot guarantee a cure, data shows it extends quality life by an average of seven years.

Informal

Colleague 1 Did you see the tray of donuts in the break room?

Colleague 2 Don't remind me! I was trying to stay strong, but I **succumbed to** / *gave in to* the temptation of the chocolate-glazed one.

Referral Letter / Discharge Summary

> During her recovery from hip surgery, the patient continued to **succumb to** / *suffer from* severe migraines that significantly impacted her rehabilitation progress. Despite aggressive treatment, the patient rapidly **succumbed to** / *died with* acute respiratory distress syndrome following admission to the ICU.

Scientific Literature

> Before the development of effective HIV antiviral therapy, the incidence and the mortality of these lymphomas was high, with patients frequently **succumbing to** the disease. Pongas, G.N., Ramos, J.C. (2022).
>
> Procrastination is a temptation to which many of us **succumb**, frequently with an impact on our wellbeing. Read, C. (2023).
>
> Poverty is a key factor in determining who will **succumb**. Stock, C. et al. (1998).

ENGLISH EXPRESSIONS IN CONTEXT

sustain (vt)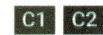

Word family: n: sustainability; adj: sustainable, sustained; adv: sustainably;
syn: maintain, uphold, suffer

to provide resources for survival; to maintain consistency over time; to endure negativity; to support an argument or theory with evidence

---

(v, adj) + n | damage | fracture, injury | growth | life | loss | recovery, stability

Dialogue

Patient   My wrist really hurts after falling off my bike this morning.

Doctor   The X-ray shows you've **sustained** / *have* (or *got, developed*) a minor **fracture** of your right radius.

Q&A

Questioner   Can you explain the sharp increase in patient enrolment during Phase 2 of your study?

Presenter   Our trial was able to **sustain** / *maintain* consistent **growth** thanks to our expanded network of participating clinics.

Informal

Colleague 1   Hey, I heard you tried that new regimen of running five miles every morning before work!

Colleague 2   Yeah, but I couldn't **sustain** / *maintain* the weight **loss** once winter came and I stopped running.

Referral Letter / Discharge Summary

> While the patient's current pain-management regimen appears effective, we need to develop a more **sustainable** / *workable* (or *lasting*) long-term treatment plan given his history of medication sensitivities.

Scientific Literature

> Patients **sustaining** an **injury** to either of these nerves must be managed correctly [...]. Loescher, A.R. et al. (2003).

> Metabolism consists of a series of reactions that occur within cells of living organisms to **sustain life**. Judge, A., Dodd, M.S. (2020).

> Understanding the complexities of establishing and sustaining recovery from substance addiction and the dynamic individual processes that occur will assist addiction treatment professionals in fostering **sustained recovery** behaviour in clients. Goshorn, J.R. et al. (2023).

MEDICAL EDITION

underscore (vt)

Word family: n: underscore; syn: underline

to highlight, emphasise or reinforce the significance or validity of something; to draw a line beneath text for emphasis

+ n | importance, relevance, point, need, significance | fact, problem | extent, value

Dialogue

Patient   I've been feeling exhausted lately, but I figured it's just stress from work.

Doctor   While stress could be a factor, your persistent fatigue **underscores** / *highlights* the **need** to check your iron levels and rule out anaemia.

Q&A

Questioner   Please could you comment on potential ethical concerns associated with the intervention?

Presenter   It's imperative to **underscore** / *emphasise* that our study strictly adhered to ethical guidelines, with careful consideration of the privacy and welfare of every participant.

Informal

Colleague 1   Have you had a chance to recap the key takeaways from the meeting?

Colleague 2   I haven't yet, but I plan to **underscore** / *highlight* the **importance** of innovation in my summary report.

Referral Letter / Discharge Summary

The attending physician **underscored** the **fact** / *emphasised* that the patient's symptoms significantly worsened when exposed to cold temperatures, which guided our subsequent treatment approach.

Scientific Literature

These findings **underscore** the **point** that the US life expectancy disadvantage originates at early age and extends across the life-course. Avendano, M., Kawachi, I. (2014).

In this study, we **underscored** the **importance** of effective crisis communication amid global health emergencies like COVID-19 [...]. Su, Z. et al. (2022).

Such diversity of diagnosis and presentation, along with therapeutic implications, **underscore** the **need** to study the profile of myocardial infarction in young persons. Gulati, R. et al. (2020).

ENGLISH EXPRESSIONS IN CONTEXT

understate (vt)

Word family: n: understatement; ant: overstate; syn: downplay

to present something as less significant, serious or severe than it actually is

+ n as object | **case** | **extent**

Dialogue

Patient My chest has been hurting for three days, but it's not too bad.

Doctor Let's not **understate** / *minimise* your **case** – your symptoms suggest a possible heart condition that requires immediate attention.

Q&A

Questioner How do you reconcile your study's favourable outcomes with the contradictory results from the Japanese lab?

Presenter I wouldn't **understate** / *minimise* the differences, but our methodology focused specifically on long-term patient outcomes rather than immediate biochemical markers.

Informal

Colleague 1 The new AI diagnostic tool seems to be getting all the buzz* at our department lately, although I'm dubious of its actual effectiveness.

Colleague 2 I wouldn't **understate** / *downplay* (or *dismiss*) its capabilities. It's actually detected three rare conditions that we initially missed.

Referral Letter / Discharge Summary

Her symptoms' severity was no **understatement** / *exaggeration*, with a Glasgow Coma Scale of 6 on admission requiring immediate ventilatory support.

Scientific Literature

The clinical significance of Epstein-Barr virus (EBV) cannot be **understated**. Sausen, D.G. et al. (2023).

Because of data limitations, complex statistical modelling is required to produce current estimates, relying on assumptions and proxies that likely **understate** the **extent** of micronutrient deficiencies and the consequent global health burden. Hess, S.Y. et al. (2021).

The recorded statistics of influenza morbidity and mortality are likely to be a significant **understatement**. Johnson, N.P., Mueller, J. (2002).

MEDICAL EDITION

uphold (vt) `C1`

to support and maintain something you consider right, ensuring its persistence; to confirm or sustain a prior decision or ruling, particularly in legal contexts

+ n as object | **principle, value, right, law** | **standard** | **reputation** |
+ n as subject | **court, judge**

Dialogue

Patient My chest has been feeling tight for a couple of days and now I'm having trouble breathing deeply.

Doctor For future reference, with such symptoms, it's important to **uphold** / *adhere to* the **principle** of timely intervention so that we can rule out any serious conditions.

Q&A

Questioner In your study, how did you ensure that ethical standards were maintained throughout the research process?

Presenter We strictly adhered to the principles outlined in the Declaration of Helsinki to **uphold** / *meet* the highest **standards** of ethical conduct in human subject research.

Informal

Colleague 1 Have you tried the local specialty coffee here?

Colleague 2 Yes, it's fantastic, and it's amazing how it **upholds** / *lives up to** the **reputation** of this region for quality beans.

Referral Letter / Discharge Summary

The nurses reported that Mr. Peterson consistently failed to **uphold** / *follow* visiting-hour policies, leading to disruption of ward routines and other patients' rest.

Scientific Literature

Under pressure, it is essential to **uphold** high bioethical **principles** and rigorous **standards** for the development and approval of medicines. No authors listed. (2020).

With the contribution of many thoughtful leaders, the Academy refreshed its commitment to promote excellence and **uphold** its high **values**. Casadevall, A. et al. (2023).

In California, gestational carrier Anna Johnson refused to give up the baby to intended parents Mark and Crispina Calvert. The couple sued her for custody (Calvert v. Johnson), and the **court upheld** their parental **rights**. Patel, N.H. et al. (2018).

ENGLISH EXPRESSIONS IN CONTEXT

visceral (adj)

Word family: n: viscera*; adv: viscerally

(literary) driven by deep emotions rather than rational thought; (anatomical) pertaining to the internal organs, especially the intestines

+ n | feeling, reaction, dislike | fat, obesity | organ

Dialogue

Patient I've been experiencing intense abdominal pain and a deep sense of unease.

Doctor Based on your symptoms and the **visceral** / *strong gut* **feeling** you've described, I suspect that there may be an underlying issue that we need to investigate further.

Q&A

Questioner Could you elaborate on the severity of the potential side effects of the new treatment?

Presenter While the side effects are generally mild, some patients may experience a **visceral reaction** / *strong negative response* to the treatment.

Informal

Colleague 1 Did you catch the keynote speech this morning? The presenter had some pretty controversial ideas.

Colleague 2 Honestly, I found myself **viscerally** / *strongly* disagreeing with many of the points they made.

Referral Letter / Discharge Summary

The patient's CT scan revealed no evidence of metastatic disease in the **visceral** / *internal* **organs**, including the liver, lungs and kidneys.

Scientific Literature

Collectively, these findings support the contention that the inherent nature of stuttered speech triggers a **visceral reaction** in a listener, irrespective of their background and knowledge about the disorder. Guntupalli, V.K. et al. (2012).

Most clinicians who participate in clinical research are **viscerally** aware that the current informed consent process is failing patients. Saylor, P.H. (2021).

Visceral fat area (VFA) is used to measure visceral obesity [...]. Liu, X. et al. (2022).

Endmatter

ENGLISH EXPRESSIONS IN CONTEXT

affect vs effect p.11

	affect	effect
transitive verb	+++ (very common)	possible but uncommon
noun	+ (in psychology)	+++ (very common)
adjective	'affective' (uncommon apart from psychology)	'effective' (very common)

'Affect' is commonly used as a transitive verb meaning 'to produce an effect upon...' and is followed by an object. In contrast, 'effect' is commonly used as a noun meaning 'result of a something' and only occasionally used as a transitive verb meaning 'to cause it to happen'. Note: 'affect' is used as a noun in psychology, meaning 'manifestations of an emotion'. Example sentence:

*The psychologist carefully observed the patient's **affect** during the therapy session.*

Although the adjective form of 'affective' is uncommon in the wider medical context, it is used in psychology – for example, 'seasonal affective disorder (SAD)', which is a type of seasonal depression.

contravene vs contradict vs controvert p.34

vt	contravene	contradict	controvert
n	contravention	contradiction	controversy
adj	contravened	contradictory	controversial
meaning/ usage	To violate, to infringe on. Most often used in reference to laws.	To say the contrary or to be directly opposed.	To engage in a dispute.
example sentences	The hospital was fined after it was found to **contravene** infection-control protocols by reusing disposable syringes.	The nurse politely corrected the patient when he **contradicted** the doctor's explanation of how insulin affects blood sugar levels.	The latest research **controverts** the long-held belief that dietary cholesterol directly contributes to heart disease.

efficiency (efficient) vs efficacy (efficacious) p.52 p.53

n	efficiency	efficacy
adj	efficient	efficacious
definition	How well resources (time, money, equipment, personnel) are used in delivering healthcare.	How well a treatment achieves its intended medical outcome.
common collocations	efficient system, efficient workflow, efficient use of resources, efficient delivery	efficacious treatment, efficacious therapy, efficacious intervention, efficacious drug
example sentences	The clinic became more **efficient** after reorganising its appointment system.	The new drug proved **efficacious** in treating depression.

evoke vs provoke p.93

	evoke	provoke
primary meaning	To bring forth or elicit something naturally.	To deliberately cause or trigger, often with negative implications.
common objects/ collocations	memories, sensations, responses, potential (in tests), emotions (neutral)	reactions, attacks, symptoms, inflammation, anger
typical medical/ scientific usage	Diagnostic contexts (e.g., evoked potentials), describing clinical observations, research findings.	Describing adverse reactions, challenge tests (e.g., provocation test), symptom triggers.
connotation	Neutral to positive; suggests natural emergence or elicitation.	Often negative; suggests deliberate instigation or aggravation.
example sentences	The scent of antiseptic can **evoke** anxiety in patients who have had traumatic hospital experiences.	Certain allergens can **provoke** a severe anaphylactic reaction in sensitive individuals.

exacerbate vs aggravate p.12 p.63

	exacerbate / exacerbation	aggravate / aggravation
primary setting	Predominantly medical and scientific documentation (research papers, clinical notes, professional communications).	Both medical and general contexts (everyday conversation, casual writing, medical documents).
formality	formal, technical	both formal and informal
typical collocations	Specifically with medical conditions, symptoms, or clinical problems (e.g., 'exacerbate asthma', 'exacerbation of COPD').	Broader range including both medical conditions and general situations (e.g., 'aggravate an injury', 'aggravate a person').
additional meanings	Single meaning: to make worse (especially medical conditions).	Multiple meanings: (1) to make worse; (2) to annoy/irritate someone; (3) legal context ('aggravating circumstances').

inference vs implication p.76

The nouns 'inference' and 'implication' frequently appear in writing, especially in scientific/medical articles. A range of dictionaries contrast the two nouns side-by-side and raise caution on their distinction. The two terms have opposite meanings. When a writer or speaker hints at something without stating it outright, they are **implying** it. On the other hand, when you draw a conclusion based on what was said, you are **inferring** it. To summarise, **inference** is 'the act of drawing a conclusion based on evidence or reasoning' whereas **implication** is 'the conclusion that can be drawn from something, even if it is not explicitly stated; to hint at something'. Examples:

- *Based on the patient's lab results, the doctor made the **inference** that the infection was viral rather than bacterial.*
- *The study's findings have serious **implications** for how we treat antibiotic-resistant infections.*

proof *vs* evidence `p.92`

'Proof' and 'evidence' have related meanings, and their difference in meaning is nuanced. In a nutshell, 'proof" is more conclusive than 'evidence'. Therefore 'proof' carries much more weight as a conclusion than 'evidence'. **Proof** is a fact that demonstrates something to be real or true, while **evidence** is information that might lead one to believe something to be real or true. Examples:

- *A biopsy provided **proof** that the tumor was malignant.*

- *Clinical trials have shown strong **evidence** that the new drug reduces mortality in heart disease patients, but more research is needed to confirm.*

remit `p.96`

as a verb	part of speech	meaning	noun form
to remit	vi	(1) To decrease in intensity or scope (regarding disease or symptoms)	remission
	vi or vt	(2) To send something such as money to someone	remittance

as a noun	part of speech	meaning	noun form
within someone's remit	British: n	Area of responsibility or authority	remit

Glossary of terms (words are denoted by an asterisk (*))

ambulation	a formal medical term that healthcare professionals use to describe a patient's ability to walk or move from place to place independently	59
antidote	substance that counteracts a poison or toxin in the body	89
ardent	very enthusiastic or passionate	10
benevolence funding	a formal term used in healthcare settings to refer to charitable or financial-assistance programmes	19
CBT	cognitive behavioural therapy	50
debt consolidation	the act of combining multiple debts into a single, larger debt that may lead to obtaining more favorable payoff terms	32
ENT	ear, nose and throat	83

equitable	(course of action) by using 'equitable', the doctor is suggesting a fair and methodical diagnostic approach that starts with testing for common, treatable causes before moving on to more complex or invasive investigations; (life) the nuance conveyed by 'equitable life' is 'a more balanced/just life', 'better living conditions' and 'life with dignity'	60
GDPR	General Data Protection Regulation	34
get all the buzz	receive widespread attention	106
hot poker	a metal rod that was traditionally used to stir or tend fireplaces or stoves	17
intrinsic factor (IF)	a glycoprotein produced in the stomach that's necessary for the absorption of vitamin B12 in the small intestine	81
IRB	Institutional Review Board	46
live up to	to meet or fulfill expectations, standards or promises	107
M. tb	Mycobacterium tuberculosis	95
polypharmacy	taking multiple medications concurrently	24
prognoses	plural of prognosis	69
RSV	Respiratory Syncytial Virus	65
scabies	contagious skin condition caused by mites	70
sciatica	nerve pain radiating down the leg	12
sundown syndrome	increased confusion and agitation in dementia patients during late afternoon/evening hours	87
viscera	the internal organs located within the body's main cavities, particularly those found in the abdominal area, such as the intestines	108

Bibliography of works cited

Abbasi, M. et al. (2024) *Pharmaceutics*. 2024 Oct 21;16(10):1344.
Aladangady, N., de, Rooy, L. (2012) *Early Human Development*. 2012 Feb;88(2):65–9.
Alimardani, V. (2021) *Drug Delivery and Translational Research*. 2021 Jun;11(3):788–816.
Alpers, D.H., Russell-Jones, G. (2013) *Biochimie*. 2013 May;95(5):989–94.
Alsayed, S.S.R., Gunosewaya, H. (2023) *International Journal of Molecular Sciences*. 2023 Mar 8;24(6):5202.
Alvarez, J. et al. (2021) *Gastroenterología y Hepatología*. 2021 Aug–Sep;44(7):519–535.
Amich, J. (2022) *Journal of Fungi*. 2022 Mar 13;8(3):295.
Amidi, A. et al. (2023) *Ugeskrift for Laeger*. 2023 Jun 26;185(26) V02230101.
Anandaiah, A., Rock, L. (2019) *Medical Teacher*. 2019 Apr;41(4):465–470.
Andring, N. et al. (2018) *Journal of Hand Surgery American Volume*. 2018 May;43(5):455–463.
Arjunan, A., Rajan, R. (2020) *Physiology & Behavior*. 2020 Dec 1;227:113136.
Aschner, M. et al. (2018) *Regulatory Toxicology and Pharmacology*. 2018 Aug;97:A1–A3.
Atkinson, A.P. et al. (2007) *Neuropsychologia*. 2007 Sep 20;45(12):2772–82.
Auchus, R.J., Chang, A.Y. (2010) *Best Practice & Research Clinical Endocrinology & Metabolism*. 2010 Apr;24(2):219–42.
Avendano, M., Kawachi, I. (2014) *Annual Review of Public Health*. 2014:35:307–25.
Aydogdu, M.O. et al. (2021) *Journal of the Royal Society Interface*. 2021 Jan;18(174):20200798.
Baier, A.W. et al. (2017) *Anesthesia & Analgesia*. 2017 Sep;125(3):952–957.
Baker, J. et al. (2022) *Journal of Smoking Cessation*. 2022 Jan 20;2022:5474397.
Balbus-Kornfeld, J.M. et al. (1995) *Occupational and Environmental Medicine*. 1995 Jan;52(1):2–12.

Balsis, S. et al. (2015) *Assessment*. 2015 Aug;22(4):399–404.
Barkovich, A.J. (2019) *Seminars in Pediatric Neurology*. 2019 Dec;32:100766.
Batrakoulis, A. et al. (2022) *Circulation: Cardiovascular Quality and Outcomes*. 2022 Jun;15(6):e008243.
Bauer, C.A. (2020) *Otolaryngologic Clinics of North America*. 2020 Aug;53(4):617–626.
Beier, M.E., Oswald, F.L. (2012) *Journal of Experimental Psychology: Applied*. 2012 Dec;18(4):331–45.
Bellussi, L.M. et al. (2023) *Multidisciplinary Respiratory Medicine*. 2023 Dec 19;18(1):939.
Beloucif, S. (2012) *Current Opinion in Anaesthesiology*. 2012 Apr;25(2):199–203.
Binagwaho, A. et al. (2022) *International Journal of Health Policy and Management*. 2022 Feb 1;11(2):100–102.
Birnie, D. et al. (2015) *Clinics in Chest Medicine*. 2015 Dec;36(4):657–68.
Black, D.W. (2001) *CNS Drugs*. 2001 Jan;15(1):17–27.
Boas, M. et al. (2006) *European Journal of Endocrinology*. 2006 May;154(5):599–611.
Boddy, L., Hiscox, J. (2016) *Microbiology Spectrum*. 2016 Dec;4(6).
Bogin, V. (2022) *Contemporary Clinical Trials Communications*. 2022 Feb 2:26:100900.
Bonney, R. et al. (2016) *Public Understanding of Science*. 2016 Jan;25(1):2–16.
Boyer, E.W. et al. (2020) *Journal of Addiction Medicine*. 2020 Dec;14(6):446–450.
Braithwaite, S., Holt-Lunstad, J. (2017) *Current Opinion in Psychology*. 2017 Feb:13:120–125.
Bridges, C. (2023) *JAMA: The Journal of the American Medical Association*. 2023 Aug 15;330(7):595–596.
Brooks, A. et al. (2012) *Global Public Health*. 2012;7(9):931–45.
Brubaker, L.T., Wilbanks, G.D. (1991) *Surgical Clinics of North America*. 1991 Oct;71(5):963–76.
Brunnauer, A. et al. (2014) *Der Nervenarzt*. 2014 Jul;85(7):811–5.
Buck, C.K. et al. (2023) *Nursing Administration Quarterly*. 2023 Jul–Sep 01;47(3):E27–E33.
Burnett, A.J. et al. (2023) *Acta Paediatrica*. 2023 Jul;112(7):1504–1510.
Buzzard, B.M. (1998) *Haemophilia*. 1998 Jul;4(4):528–31.
Byrnes, M.C. et al. (2005) *American Journal of Surgery*. 2005 Mar;189(3):310–4.
Böckerman, P. et al. (2009) *Social Science & Medicine*. 2008 Mar;66(6):1346–55.
Bø, K., Nygaard, I.E. (2020) *Sports Medicine*. 2020 Mar;50(3):471–484.
Cadet, M.J. (2020) *Workplace Health & Safety*. 2020 Dec;68(12):583.
Cargill, T., Barnes, E. (2021) *Clinical & Experimental Immunology*. 2021 Aug;205(2):106–118.
Casadevall, A. et al. (2023) *mBio*. 2023 Dec 19;14(6):e0233423.
Chagin, A.S., Sävendahl, L. (2007) *Pediatric Endocrinology Reviews*. 2007 Jun;4(4):329–34.
Chahine, L.M. et al. (2023) *Journal of Parkinson's Disease*. 2023;13(3):297–309.
Chandrashekar, H. et al. (2019) *Indian Journal of Psychiatry*. 2019 Apr;61(Suppl 4):S724–S729.
Cheng, Z. et al. (2022) *International Journal of Environmental Research and Public Health*. 2022 Sep 28;19(19):12371.
Chiruta, C. et al. (2013) *Bioorganic & Medicinal Chemistry*. 2013 May 15;21(10):2733–41.
Chisti, Y. (2007) *Biotechnology Advances*. 2007 May–Jun;25(3):294–306.
Cho, H. et al. (2020) *Communications Biology*. 2020 Oct 1;3(1):547.
Cleveland, K.C. et al. (2016) *Journal of Applied Developmental Psychology*. 2016 Mar–Apr;43:1–7.
Cochrane, B.A. et al. (2021) *Attention, Perception, & Psychophysics*. 2021 Jan;83(1):58–66.
Cohen, J.J. (2003) *Journal of the American Medical Association*. 2003 Mar 5;289(9):1143–9.
Coldiron, B.M. (1996) *Dermatologic Surgery*. 1996 Mar;22(3):296–9.
Contini, P., Osmanaj, E. (2023) *Frontiers in Sociology*. 2023 Oct 19;8:1111690.
Conway, M.J. et al. (2023) *Viruses*. 2023 Feb 8;15(2):469.
Crevel, R.W. et al. (2000) *Food and Chemical Toxicology*. 2000 Apr;38(4):385–93.
Cromby, J. (2012) *Journal of Health Psychology*. 2012 Oct;17(7):943–57.
Cummings, K.M. et al. (2007) *Cancer Epidemiology, Biomarkers & Prevention*. 2007 Jun;16(6):1070–6.
Dalan, R. et al. (2022) *Frontiers in Endocrinology*. 2022 Jul 6:13:943993.
Daruwalla, K., Lipasti, M. (2024) *Frontiers in Computational Neuroscience*. 2024 May 16;18:1240348.
Darveaux, J.I., Lemanske, J.R.R.F. (2014) *Journal of Allergy and Clinical Immunology: In Practice*. 2014 Nov–Dec;2(6):658–63.
Dawson, M.A., Kouzarides, T. (2012) *Cell*. 2012 Jul 6;150(1):12–27.

De Souza Valente, C. (2022) *Veterinary and Animal Science*. 2022 May 14;16:100252.
Deng, Q. et al. (2020) *International Journal of Cardiology*. 2020 Jul 15;311:116–121.
Dhaliwal, R. et al. (2022) *Journal of Clinical Endocrinology & Metabolism*. 2022 Apr 19;107(5):1205–1215.
Dhama, K. et al. (2020) *Clinical Microbiology Reviews*. 2020 Jun 24;33(4):e00028–20.
Diamond, A. (2006) *Trends in Cognitive Sciences*. 2006 May;10(5):212–8.
Dolk, H. et al. (2010) *Advances in Experimental Medicine and Biology*. 2010;686:349–64.
Dominiak, Ł. (2024) *Journal of Bioethical Inquiry*. 2024 Sep 24. doi: 10.1007/s11673-024-10374-8. Online ahead of print.
Donny, E.C. et al. (2014) *Preventive Medicine*. 2014 Nov;68:17–22.
Dopytalska, K. et al. (2018) *Reumatologia*. 2018;56(6):392–398.
Douglas, C.W. et al. (1990) *FEMS Microbiology Letters*. 1990 Oct;60(1–2):63–7.
Dowd, A. (2023) *Methods in Molecular Biology*. 2023;2596:421–428.
Dwyer, G. et al. (2022) *The American Naturalist*. 2022 Jan;199(1):108–125.
Edridge, A.W.D., van der Hoek, L. (2020) *PLoS Neglected Tropical Diseases*. 2020 Oct 28;14(10):e0008856.
Eiden, M. et al. (2006) *Journal of Veterinary Medicine, Series B: Infectious Diseases and Veterinary Public Health*. 2006 Aug;53(6):251–6.
Einarson, T.R. et al. (2012) *Journal of Population Therapeutics and Clinical Pharmacology*. 2012;19(2):e334–48.
Ero, R. et al. (2019) *Protein Science*. 2019 Apr;28(4):684–693.
Escobar-Bravo, R. et al. (2017) *Frontiers in Plant Science*. 2017 Mar 2;8:278.
Ettinger, D., Jehiel, P. (2021) *Experimental Economics*. 2021;24(3):821–853.
Fang, Z. et al. (2021) *International Journal of Ophthalmology*. 2021 Sep 18;14(9):1310–1314.
Farage, M.A. (2012) *Global Journal of Health Science*. 2012 Feb 29;4(2):2–25.
Fareri, D.S. (2019) *Frontiers in Human Neuroscience*. 2019 Aug 13;13:271.
Fassin, Y. (2021) *Scientometrics*. 2021;126(6):5305–5319.
Feng, S. et al. (2023) *Nature Communications*. 2023 Aug 12;14(1):4874.
Flor, H. (2002) *The Lancet Neurology*. 2002 Jul;1(3):182–9.
Foda, H.M.T. (2005) *Plastic and Reconstructive Surgery*. 2005 Feb;115(2):406–15.
Foel, O.F. et al. (2020) *Plastic and Reconstructive Surgery Global Open*. 2020 May 21;8(5):e2849.
Fricchione, G., Beach, S. (2019) *Handbook of Clinical Neurology*. 2019;166:223–252.
Fridlind, A.M. et al. (2004) *Science*. 2004 Apr 30;304(5671):718–22.
Friston, K. (2023) *Molecular Psychiatry*. 2023 Jan;28(1):256–268.
Fry, M. (2007) *Frontiers in Bioscience*. 2007 May 1;12:4336–51.
Fuchs, M.M., Connolly, H.M. (2020) *Cardiology Clinics*. 2020 Aug;38(3):353–363.
Fürstenau, M. et al. (2024) *The Lancet Oncology*. 2024 Jun;25(6):744–759.
Galea, L.A. et al. (2009) *Journal of Plastic, Reconstructive & Aesthetic Surgery*. 2009 Jun;62(6):737–41.
Garcia, M.B. et al. (2020) *Advances in Experimental Medicine and Biology*. 2020;1257:193–207.
Gardiner, F.W. (2016) *Annals of Medicine and Surgery*. 2016 Jul 13;10:19–21.
Gattinoni, L. et al. (2015) *Critical Care*. 2015;19 Suppl 3(Suppl 3):S7.
Ghasemian, A., Christakis, N.A. (2023) *Scientific Reports*. 2023 Nov 16;13(1):20040.
Gill, P. et al. (2003) *Forensic Science International*. 2003 Jan 28;131(2–3):184–96.
Givi, B. et al. (2020) *JAMA Otolaryngology–Head & Neck Surgery*. 2020 Jun 1;146(6):579–584.
Golding, J.F., Gresty, M.A. *Current Opinion in Neurology*. 2005 Feb;18(1):29–34.
Goma, A.A., Phillips, C.J.C. (2022) *Animals*. 2022 Jul 29;12(15):1937.
Gonzalez, C.G. et al. (2022) *Oncology Letters*. 2022 Mar;23(3):74.
González, F. et al. (2021) *Molecules*. 2021 Jul 1;26(13):4042.
Goo, H.W. (2021) *Korean Journal of Radiology*. 2021 Sep;22(9):1441–1450.
Goodwin, G.P., Gromet, D.M. (2014) *Wiley Interdisciplinary Reviews: Cognitive Science*. 2014 Sep;5(5):561–572.
Gorchein, A. (1997) *The Lancet*. 1997 Oct 11;350(9084):1104.
Goshorn, J.R. et al. (2023) *Substance Use & Misuse*. 2023;58(7):900–909.
Graham, D.Y. (2024) *Current Topics in Microbiology and Immunology*. 2024;445:127–154.
Greenfield, S. (1998) *Essays in Biochemistry*. 1998;33:179–91.

Grobusch, M.P. et al. (2020) *Travel Medicine and Infectious Disease*. 2020 Nov–Dec:38:101753.
Grossman, E., Messerli, F.H. (2012) *American Journal of Medicine*. 2012 Jan;125(1):14–22.
Gruber, R.P. et al. (2018) *Hals-Nasen-Ohrenheilkunde*. 2018 Jan;66(1):26–31.
Gulati, R. et al. (2020) *Mayo Clinic Proceedings*. 2020 Jan;95(1):136–156.
Guntupalli, V.K. et al. (2012) *International Journal of Language & Communication Disorders*. 2012 Sep–Oct;47(5):603–8.
Guyotte, K.W. et al. (2023) *Women's Studies International Forum*. 2023 May–Jun;98:102755.
Halson, S.L. (2014) *Sports Medicine*. 2014 May;44 Suppl 1(Suppl 1):S13–23.
Han, X. et al. (2023) *Seminars in Liver Disease*. 2023 Nov;43(4):383–401.
Hauw, F. et al. (2023) *Cortex*. 2023 Mar:160:167–179.
Hawley, A. et al. (2019) *Wilderness and Environmental Medicine*. 2019 Mar;30(1):44–51.
Heaton, H.A. et al. (2020) *Emergency Medicine Journal*. 2020 Sep;37(9):552–554.
Hedlund, C.S. (1991) *Problems in Veterinary Medicine*. 1991 Jun;3(2):198–209.
Hegeman, M.A. et al. (2011) *British Journal of Pharmacology*. 2011 Jul;163(5):1048–58.
Helbok, R. et al. (2022) *Neurocritical Care*. 2022 Aug;37(1):47–59.
Hess, S.Y. et al. (2021) *Current Developments in Nutrition*. 2021 Nov 18;5(12):nzab141.
Hintze, A., Hertwig, R. (2016) *Scientific Reports*. 2016 Sep 28:6:34102.
Ho, P.M. et al. (2006) *Archives of Internal Medicine*. 2006 Sep 25;166(17):1836–41.
Hodgson, A., Park, K.J. (2019) *Archives of Pathology & Laboratory Medicine*. 2019 Jan;143(1):34–46.
Holstein, S.A. et al. (2023) *Journal of Clinical Oncology*. 2023 Sep 20;41(27):4416–4429.
Hu, Y. (2019) *Infection and Drug Resistance*. 2019 Sep 27:12:3063–3066.
Huet, A.C. et al. (2022) *Analytical and Bioanalytical Chemistry*. 2022 Mar;414(8):2553–2570.
Humphreys, I.M., Hwang, P.H. (2015) *Otolaryngologic Clinics of North America*. 2015 Oct;48(5):871–81.
Hussein, M.R. (2013) *Expert Review of Hematology*. 2013 Dec;6(6):713–33.
Ilgaya, K. et al. (2019) *Nature Communications*. 2019 Apr 1;10(1):1466.
Ilyas, M. (2017) *Pathobiology*. 2017;84(6):292–305.
Ishijima, T., Nakajima, K. (2023) *Biology*. 2023 Aug 11;12(8):1121.
Jacobson, R.M. et al. (2015) *Mayo Clinic Proceedings*. 2015 Nov;90(11):1562–8.
Jassim, A. et al. (2023) *Nature Reviews Cancer*. 2023 Oct;23(10):710–724.
Jeffery, K.J. (2023) *Philosophical Transactions of the Royal Society B: Biological Sciences*. 2023 Jan 30;378(1869):20210452.
Jetté, N. et al. (2016) *The Lancet Neurology*. 2016 Aug;15(9):982–994.
Johanson, G. (2020) *International Journal of Hygiene and Environmental Health*. 2020 May;226:113488.
Johnson, N.P., Mueller, J. (2002) *Bulletin of the History of Medicine*. 2002 Spring;76(1):105–15.
Jones, D.R. (1992) *Journal of the Royal Society of Medicine*. 1992 Mar;85(3):165–8.
Jordan, S.C., Pescovitz, M.D. (2006) *Clinical Journal of the American Society of Nephrology*. 2006 May;1(3):421–32.
Judge, A., Dodd, M.S. (2020) *Essays in Biochemistry*. 2020 Oct 8;64(4):607–647.
Junginger, J. et al. (1998) *Psychiatric Services*. 1998 Feb;49(2):218–20.
Jönsson, L. et al. (2024) *Alzheimer's Research & Therapy*. 2024 Feb 29;16(1):48.
Kanazawa, K. (1990) *Japanese Journal of Geriatrics*. 1990 Mar;27(2):129–31.
Karp, C. et al. (2024) *BMC Pregnancy and Childbirth*. 2024 Jan 3;24(1):21.
Karrer, W. (2005) *Swiss Medical Weekly*. 2005 Feb 5;135(5–6):71–5.
Keller, R.G., Patel, K.G. (2015) *Facial Plastic Surgery Clinics of North America*. 2015 Aug;23(3):373–92.
Keller, J.M. (2019) *The Journal of Sexual Medicine*. 2019 May;16(5):618–620.
Kelly, L.J., Khemlani, S. (2023) *Journal of Experimental Psychology: General*. 2023 Jun;152(6):1639–1646.
Kelly, J.P. (2022) *British Medical Journal*. 2022 Feb 24:376:o476.
Kennedy, M.S. (2018) *American Journal of Nursing*. 2018 Sep;118(9):7.
Khorasani, A.M. et al. (2000) *Journal of Andrology*. 2000 Jul–Aug;21(4):586–94.
Kiani, A.K. (2022) *Journal of Preventive Medicine and Hygiene*. 2022 Oct 17;63(2 Suppl 3):E255–E266.
Kimmel, K. et al. (2023) *Nature Ecology & Evolution*. 2023 Sep;7(9):1525–1536.
Klebanov, L.B., Yakovlev, A.Y. (2008) *Biology Direct*. 2008 Aug 20:3:35.

Koolhaas, J.M. et al. (2016) *Neurobiology of Stress*. 2016 Sep 23:6:104–112.
Korsgaard, S., Schmidt (2024) *Ugeskrift for Laeger*. 2024 Apr 8;186(15):V12230789.
Kumar, S. et al. (2012) *BMC Nephrology*. 2012 Sep 10:13:107.
Lang, J. (2020) *Current Opinion in Psychology*. 2020 Oct:35:17–20.
Langer, E.J., Imber, L.G. (1979) *Journal of Personality and Social Psychology*. 1979 Nov;37(11):2014–24.
Lee, M.C.C., Ding, A.Y.L. (2024) *Psychological Reports*. 2024 Apr;127(2):887–911.
Levin, M.G., Burgess, S. (2024) *JAMA Cardiology*. 2024 Jan 1;9(1):79–89.
Levin, M.G., Burgess, S. (2024) *JAMA Cardiology*. 2024 Jan 1;9(1):79–89.
León-Menjivar, C.D. (2022) *Hispanic Health Care International*. 2022 Sep;20(3):195–201.
Li, X., Atkinson, M.A. (2015) *Pediatric Diabetes*. 2015 Nov;16(7):485–92.
Li, L. et al. (2022) *Frontiers in Public Health*. 2022 May 19:10:791977.
Liao, C.C. et al. (2021) *Journal of Obstetrics and Gynaecology*. 2021 Jan;41(1):21–31.
Lickliter, R. (2017) *Wiley Interdisciplinary Reviews: Cognitive Science*. 2017 Jan;8(1–2).
Liu, L. et al. (2023) *Journal of Inflammation Research*. 2023 Jul 1;16:2727–2754.
Liu, D.Q. et al. (2019) *Current Neuropharmacology*. 2019;17(4):366–376.
Liu, X. et al. (2022) *Frontiers in Oncology*. 2022 Sep 20:12:957527.
Loescher, A.R. et al. (2003) *Dental Update*. 2003 Sep;30(7):375–80, 382.
Loomba, R. et al. (2023) *The Lancet Gastroenterology & Hepatology*. 2023 Jun;8(6):511–522.
Low, K.J.Y. et al. (2021) *Journal of Advanced Research*. 2021 May 20:36:113–132.
Lowewenstein et al. (2001) *Psychological Bulletin*. 2001 Mar;127(2):267–86.
Luengo, O., Cardona, V. (2014) *Clinical and Translational Allergy*. 2014 Sep 8:4:28.
Lundin, L., Flyckt, L. (2015) *Läkartidningen*. 2015 Oct 13:112:DHI7.
Lutz, C.T. et al. (2011) *Journal of Immunology*. 2011 Apr 15;186(8):4590–8.
Ma, C. et al. (2019) *Drugs*. 2019 Aug;79(12):1321–1335.
Machado, S. et al. (2009) *Arquivos de Neuro-Psiquiatria*. 2009 Jun;67(2A):334–42.
Magnan, J. et al. (2018) *Journal of International Advanced Otology*. 2018 Aug;14(2):317–321.
Malik, A.A. et al. (2020) *Science Robotics*. 2020 Jun 17;5(43):eabc2782.
Mandal, J. et al. (2016) *Tropical Parasitology*. 2016 Jan–Jun;6(1):5–7.
March, P.A. (1996) *Veterinary Clinics of North America: Small Animal Practice*. 1996 Jul;26(4):945–71.
Mascaro, O., Kovács, Á.M. (2022) *Developmental Science*. 2022 Jul;25(4):e13223.
Matte, A. et al. (2023) *Current Opinion in Hematology*. 2023 May 1;30(3):93–98.
Maughan, R.J. (1995) *International Journal of Sport Nutrition*. 1995 Jun;5(2):94–101.
McAllum, K. et al. (2021) *Research on Aging*. 2021 Aug;43(7–8):263–273.
McFarlane, J. (1989) *Women & Health*. 1989;15(3):69–84.
Middleton, S. (2010) *Veterinary Clinics of North America: Food Animal Practice*. 2010 Nov;26(3):557–72.
Mitra, S. (2023) *European Journal of Preventive Cardiology*. 2023 Sep 6;30(12):1289–1290.
Mohajir, W.A. et al. (2022) *Medical Clinics of North America*. 2022 Sep;106(5S):e1–e16.
Mohammed, A. et al. (2021) *Nature Reviews Immunology*. 2021 Dec;21(12):823–828.
Moore, P.C. et al. (2023) *Advances in Cancer Research*. 2023;158:1–39.
Mu, A. et al. (2021) *BMC Geriatrics*. 2021 Apr 21;21(1):264.
Murota, H., Katayama, I. (2017) *Allergology International*. 2017 Jan;66(1):8–13.
Murphy, G. et al. (2023) *PLOS ONE*. 2023 Jul 6;18(7):e0287503.
Naeem, B.S., Bhatti (2020) *Health Information and Libraries Journal*. 2020 Sep;37(3):233–239.
Narasimhan, M. et al. (2019) *British Medical Journal*. 2019 Apr 1;365:l1403.
Nasr-Esfahani, M.H. et al. (2012) *International Journal of Andrology*. 2012 Aug;35(4):475–84.
Nava, E. et al. (2017) *Frontiers in Psychology*. 2017 Nov 15;8:1994.
Neufeld, M. (2021) *Prospects*. 2021;51(1–3):175–184.
Nickel, B. et al. (2021) *BMJ Open*. 2021 Aug 18;11(8):e047513.
No authors listed. (2020) *Nature Cancer*. 2020;1(9):855–856.
No authors listed. (2019) *World Health Organization Guidelines for Malaria Vector Control*. Geneva: World Health Organization; 2019.
Noorbakhsh, J. et al. (2020) *Molecular Cancer Research*. 2020 Jan;18(1):20–26.
Nwadiugwu, M.C. (2020) *Journal of Aging Research*. 2020 Jun 29;2020:6759521.
Oates, G.R. et al. (2020) *American Journal of Health Behavior*. 2020 Mar 1;44(2):232–243.

Ogunleye, T.A. (2023) *Dermatologic Clinics*. 2023 Apr;41(2):285–290.
Olingy, C.E. et al. (2019) *Journal of Leukocyte Biology*. 2019 Aug;106(2):309–322.
Oliva, J. (2019) *International Journal of Molecular Sciences*. 2019 Nov 5;20(21):5511.
Oudesluys-Murphy, A.M. et al. (1996) *European Journal of Pediatrics*. 1996 Jun;155(6):429–35.
O'Leary, K.D., Woodin, E.M. (2005) *Clinical Psychology Review*. 2005 Nov;25(7):877–94.
Pabis, M. et al. (2011) *Journal of Advanced Nursing*. 2011 Feb;67(2):384–93.
Pajic-Lijakovic, I., Milivojevic, M. (2023) *European Biophysics Journal*. 2023 Feb;52(1–2):1–15.
Pal, S. et al. (2015) *Nutrients*. 2015 Aug 31;7(9):7285–97.
Paling, C. (2021) *Musculoskeletal Science and Practice*. 2021 Aug:54:102379.
Pallas, V., Garcia, J.A. (2011) *Journal of General Virology*. 2011 Dec;92(Pt 12):2691–2705.
Panigrahi, A. et al. (2014) *BioMed Research International*. 2014:2014:979827.
Patel, N.H. et al. (2018) *Journal of Human Reproduction Sciences*. 2018 Jul–Sep;11(3):212–218.
Penn, J.L., Deutsch, C. (2022) *Science*. 2022 Apr 29;376(6592):524–526.
Pennycook, G., Rand, D.G. (2021) *Trends in Cognitive Sciences*. 2021 May;25(5):388–402.
Pfeifer, I. et al. (2016) *Placenta*. 2016 Jan:37:56–60.
Platt, B., Riedel, G. (2011) *Behavioural Brain Research*. 2011 Aug 10;221(2):499–504.
Poddubnyy, D. (2020) *Rheumatology*. 2020 Oct 1;59(Suppl4):iv6–iv17.
Polak, T.B. et al. (2022) *BMJ Open*. 2022 Apr 8;12(4):e058279.
Pongas, G.N., Ramos, J.C. (2022) *Journal of Clinical Medicine*. 2022 Mar 7;11(5):1447.
Prasad, V. et al. (2016) *The Lancet Oncology*. 2016 Feb;17(2):e81–e86.
Price, A. et al. (2022) *Campbell Systematic Reviews*. 2022 Jul 26;18(3):e1264.
Purcell, B.A., Palmeri, T.J. (2017) *Journal of Mathematical Psychology*. 2017 Feb;76(B):156–171.
Querido, J.B. et al. (2024) *Nature Reviews Molecular Cell Biology*. 2024 Mar;25(3):168–186.
Rattenborg, N.C., Ungurean, G. (2022) *Trends in Ecology & Evolution*. 2023 Feb;38(2):156–170.
Read, C. (2023) *Veterinary Record*. 2023 Feb;192(4):180–181.
Resnik, D.B., Finn, P.R. (2018) *Science and Engineering Ethics*. 2018 Aug;24(4):1241–1252.
Retrouvey, H., Gdalevitch, P. (2018) *Plastic Surgery*. 2018 Aug;26(3):145–147.
Reynolds, D. (2006) *Holistic Nursing Practice*. 2006 May–Jun;20(3):118–21.
Richburg, C.E. et al. (2023) *Surgical Clinics of North America*. 2023 Apr;103(2):271–285.
Rindflesh, T.C. et al. (2017) *ILAR Journal*. 2017 Jul 1;58(1):80–89.
Risen, J.L. (2016) *Psychological Review*. 2016 Mar;123(2):182–207.
Rivlin, K. et al. (2024) *JAMA Network Open*. 2024 Aug 1;7(8):e2426248.
Rizkallah, J. et al. (2009) *Chest*. 2009 Mar;135(3):786–793.
Robine, J., Vaupel, J.W. (2001) *Experimental Gerontology*. 2001 Apr;36(4–6):915–30.
Rodd, B.G. et al. (2022) *Critical Reviews in Food Science and Nutrition*. 2022;62(26):7354–7369.
Romaguera, A. et al. (2017) *CNS & Neurological Disorders Drug Targets*. 2017;16(5):592–597.
Rosu-Finsen (2023) *Nature Reviews Chemistry*. 2023 Feb;7(2):72.
Rothstein, M.A. (2023) *Clinical Obstetrics and Gynecology*. 2023 Jun 1;66(2):267–277.
Ru, X. et al. (2020) *Frontiers in Physiology*. 2020 Apr 2:11:283.
Ryu, H.S., Choi, S.C. (2015) *Intestinal Research*. 2015 Oct;13(4):297–305.
Sausen, D.G. et al. (2023) *Cancers*. 2023 Apr 4;15(7):2133.
Saylor, P.J. (2021) *The Oncologist*. 2021 Nov;26(11):902–903.
Schattner, A. (2021) *American Journal of Medicine*. 2021 Apr;134(4):435–443.e5.
Schichtel, M. et al. *Journal of General Internal Medicine*. 2020 Mar;35(3):874–884.
Schoppe, K.A. (2017) *Journal of the American College of Radiology*. 2017 May;14(5):714–715.
Scurria, S. et al. (2019) *Journal of Legal Medicine*. 2019 Jan–Mar;39(1):35–53.
Segall, M. et al. (2015) *Drug Discovery Today*. 2015 Sep;20(9):1093–103.
Serio, T.R. (2016) *Molecular Biology of the Cell*. 2016 Nov 1;27(21):3192–3193.
Shah, M. (2017) *Cardiology in the Young*. 2017 Jan;27(S1):S25–S30.
Shaham, G., Aviezer, H. (2022) *Emotion*. 2022 Jun;22(4):641–652.
Shamardani, K., Monje, M. (2023) *Cancer Cell*. 2023 Sep 11;41(9):1541–1543.
Shemesh, C.S. et al. (2021) *Molecular Therapy*. 2021 Feb 3;29(2):555–570.
Shi, L. et al. (2020) *The Lancet Planetary Health*. 2020 Dec;4(12):e557–e565.
Shi, Y. et al. (2022) *ACS Synthetic Biology*. 2022 Apr 15;11(4):1497–1509.
Shiga, T. et al. (2011) *NeuroReport*. 2011 May 11;22(7):337–41.
Shively, E.H. et al. (1990) *American Journal of Surgery*. 1990 Apr;159(4):380–4; discussion 385.
Smith, A.N. (2014) *Veterinary Clinics of North America: Small Animal Practice*. 2014 Sep;44(5):965–75.

Smith, P.H. et al. (1995) *Women's Health*. 1995 Winter;1(4):273–88.
Snow, M.D. et al. (2023) *Psychiatry, Psychology and Law*. 2023 Apr 20;31(2):179–188.
Sogunro, R. (1993) *Santé en Salud*. 1993 Summer;(2):5–6.
Spalding, R. (2021) *Applied Psychology: Health and Well-Being*. 2021 Feb;13(1):3–33.
Spinu, N. (2022) *Computational Toxicology*. 2022 Feb:21:100205.
Staresina, B.P. (2024) *Trends in Cognitive Sciences*. 2024 Apr;28(4):339–351.
Stock, C. et al. (1998) *Work: A Journal of Prevention, Assessment & Rehabilitation*. 1998;10(1):85–99.
Stoumpos, A.I. et al. (2023) *International Journal of Environmental Research and Public Health*. 2023 Feb 15;20(4):3407.
Streeck, H. (2016) *Current Opinion in HIV and AIDS*. 2016 Nov;11(6):593–600.
Su, Z. et al. (2022) *Frontiers in Public Health*. 2022 Nov 22:10:796572.
Sun, R., Zhao, Y. (2023) *Journal of Mathematical Economics*. 2023 Mar:105:102819.
Tak, Y.W. et al. (2022) *Journal of Korean Medical Science*. 2022 Jul 4;37(26):e205.
Takegaki, J. et al. (2019) *Biochemical and Biophysical Research Communications*. 2019 Nov 26;520(1):73–78.
Taverna, D.M., Goldstein, R.A. (2002) *Journal of Molecular Biology*. 2002 Jan 18;315(3):479–84.
Teufel, C., Fletcher, P.C. (2020) *Nature Reviews Neuroscience*. 2020 Apr;21(4):231–242.
Tian, H. et al. (2021) *Cell Stress & Chaperones*. 2021 Mar;27(2):149–164.
Tonosaki, K. et al. (2007) *Biomedical Research*. 2007 Apr;28(2):79–83.
Ushach, I., Zlotnik, A. (2016) *Journal of Leukocyte Biology*. 2016 Sep;100(3):481–9.
Uysal, C.A., Ertas, N.M. (2017) *Journal of Craniofacial Surgery*. 2017 Nov;28(8):e793.
van Luijtelaar, G. et al. (2014) *Advances in Experimental Medicine and Biology*. 2014:813:81–91.
van Spronsen, F.J. et al. (2017) *Advances in Experimental Medicine and Biology*. 2017;959:197–204.
Varelius, J. (2019) *Bioethics*. 2019 Jan;33(1):195–200.
Venney, C.J. et al. (2024) *Genome Biology and Evolution*. 2024 Feb 1;16(2):evae013.
Vento, S. (2023) *The Lancet*. 2023 Jan 28;401(10373):267–268.
Verdonk, P. et al. (2014) *BMC Medical Education*. 2014 May 17;14:96.
Verdú-Delgado, M. (2004) *Gaceta Sanitaria*. 2004 May;18 Suppl 1:118–25.
Vongraviopap, S., Asawanonda, P. (2016) *International Journal of Dermatology*. 2016 May;55(5):587–91.
Vora, D. et al. (2022) *Pharmaceutics*. 2022 Mar 20;14(3):680.
Wang, R. et al. (2019) *Frontiers in Cellular and Infection Microbiology*. 2019 May 8:9:147.
Waterman, Y.R., Peeters, M.G. (2004) *International Journal of Occupational and Environmental Health*. 2004 Apr–Jun;10(2):166–76.
Wei, F.L. et al. (2021) *International Journal of Surgery*. 2021 Jan;85:19–28.
Wei, Y. et al. (2024) *Nature Reviews Microbiology*. 2024 Nov;22(11):705–721.
Wells, E. (2017) *Journal of Medical Biography*. 2017 Nov;25(4):222–226.
Western, M.J., Nordberg, A. (2022) *Nurse Leader*. 2022 Apr;20(2):174–178.
Wiles, L. (1991) *British Dental Journal*. 1991 Nov 23;171(10):304–5.
Wilkinson, M.D. (1989) *British Dental Journal*. 1989 Apr 22;166(8):299–302.
Willet, W.C. et al. (1983) *The Lancet*. 1983 Jul 16;2(8342):130–4.
Williams, D.R., Mohammed, S.A. (2009) *Journal of Behavioral Medicine*. 2009 Feb;32(1):20–47.
Williams, L.M. et al. (2015) *NeuroImage*. 2009 Sep;47(3):804–14.
Willsteed, E. et al. (2017) *Science of The Total Environment*. 2017 Jan 15:577:19–32.
Wiseman, K.C. (1991) *ANNA Journal*. 1991 Oct;18(5):469–78, 504.
Wojtak, A., Stuart, N. (2023) *Healthcare Quarterly*. 2023 Oct;26(3):1–3.
Wolf, J.B.W., Ellegren, H. (2017) *Nature Reviews Genetics*. 2017 Feb;18(2):87–100.
Woolf, S.H., George, J.N. (2000) *Hematology/Oncology Clinics of North America*. 2000 Aug;14(4):761–84.
Yaden, D.B. et al. (2021) *PLOS ONE*. 2021 Apr 14;16(4):e0249193.
Youngster, I. et al. (2010) *Drug Safety*. 2010 Sep 1;33(9):713–26.
Zachar, P., Kendler, K.S. (2017) *Annual Review of Clinical Psychology*. 2017 May 8;13:49–71.
Zeelenberg, R. et al. (2003) *Psychonomic Bulletin & Review*. 2003 Sep;10(3):653–60.
Zhang, B. et al. (2023) *European Journal of Nutrition*. 2023 Mar;62(2):573–588.

Zhang, B. et al. (2023) *JAMA Network Open*. 2023 Sep 5;6(9):e2333470.
Zhao, F. et al. (2023) *Computers in Biology and Medicine*. 2023 Oct;165:107391.
Zheng, Z. et al. (2022) *Frontiers in Immunology*. 2022 Feb 17;13:849050.
Zhivago, K.A. et al. (2020) *Frontiers in Aging Neuroscience*. 2020 Nov 19;12:576922.
Zoltowski, B.D. et al. (2019) *Proceedings of the National Academy of Sciences of the United States of America*. 2019 Sep 24;116(39):19449–19457.
Zvidzayi, M. et al. (2021) *Pharmaceutics*. 2021 Sep 13;13(9):1456.

Also available

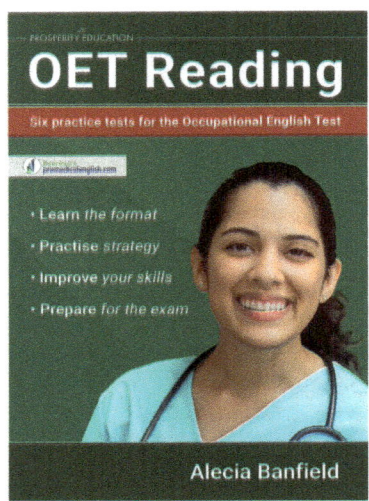

Six Reading tests (Parts A–C) with answer keys, providing a large bank of high-quality practice material for students preparing for the Occupational English Test (OET) Reading sub-test.

Practice makes perfect...

The different kinds of textual content and layout presented in the OET Reading paper require candidates to not only be confident in their control of language but also proficiently display a range of strategies and skills for parts A, B and C.

This edition of sample tests has been written to closely replicate the OET exam experience, and has undergone rigorous expert and peer review. Students will appreciate the wide range of practical and relevant texts, and benefit from the repetitive practice, something that is key to preparing for this part of the examination.

Dr. Alecia Banfield (MBBS, MPH, TEFL/TESOL) is a Medical English specialist and a certified OET Premium Preparation Partner who has helped thousands of healthcare professionals achieve exam success.

Download a **free sample test** from www.prosperityeducation.net

www.ingramcontent.com/pod-product-compliance
Lightning Source LLC
Chambersburg PA
CBHW061150070526
44584CB00034B/4472